"Dipika shares honestly and tend [...] ence, the anatomy of the feminir [...] profound expression of Ayurveda, especially in this field. It's the panacea to a modern woman's vitality through their many phases of life. What a gift this book is to womankind, and to those men, like myself, who would know women more deeply."

TIM MITCHELL, International Vedic teacher of Meditation, Ayurveda, and Yoga

"Every woman truly wishing to live all stages of their womanhood with self-love and wellness need to read this book. Dipika embodies a vast, deep wisdom of Ayurveda and the divine feminine that are shared eloquently and will empower you. This book is a legacy to all women."

DR. SMITA NARAM, founder of Ayushakti Ayurved Corporation and Global Health Centers

"All women yearning to navigate all phases of their womanhood with masterful grace need to read this book! Dipika's deep wisdom of Ayurveda will inspire you to create simple self-care routines that will reveal your most vital feminine radiance at any age."

ANANDRA GEORGE, author of *Mantra Yoga* and founder of Heart of Sound and True Freedom Coaching

"Dipika is *The* Ayurvedic Woman! She shares with the resounding pulse of the divine feminine... This book is... a must read."

JANET BRAY ATTWOOD, *New York Times*–bestselling author of *The Passion Test* and *Your Hidden Riches*

"This book is an inspiring message to all women who want to connect to their feminine nature and reclaim their strength and vitality! Dipika does a fabulous job making this ancient wisdom accessible to all women living in these modern times."

DR. MANISHA KSHIRSAGAR, BAMS (Ayu-India), Director of the Ayurveda Healing Institute and author of *Enchanting Beauty*

"Dipika is a beautiful soul, healer, and teacher. In this elegant book, she shares her knowledge, deep wisdom, and experience to guide women in the healing power of Ayurvedic lifestyle. For vibrant health, we must all live in accord with our inner nature and outer nature, which are one and the same. Ayurveda shows us how."

NANCY LONSDORF, MD, Maharishi Ayurveda and Functional Medicine physician and author of *The Healthy Brain Solution for Women over Forty* and *The Ageless Woman*. www.drnancyhealth.com.

"For over forty years, Ayurvedic practices have been an indispensable part of my daily routine. In fact, I attribute my own unlimited physical energy and strength, mental clarity, and inner tranquility to these practices. In *The Ayurvedic Woman*, Dipika clearly and eloquently shares how you too can easily incorporate Ayurveda into your own routine so that you can enjoy a long, healthy, and vibrant life. This book is a true gift to all women."

DEBRA PONEMAN, motivational speaker and founder of Yes to Success Seminars, Inc.

"Dipika Delmenico eloquently shares her profound knowledge of Ayurveda and vast, deep wisdom about the divine feminine in this beautiful book. If you want greater self-love and empowerment, dive into these pages."

MARCI SHIMOFF, #1 *New York Times*–bestselling author of *Happy for No Reason* and *Chicken Soup for the Woman's Soul*

The Ayurvedic Woman

THE
Ayurvedic
Woman

The Essential Guide for **Wellness** in All Phases of **Womanhood**

DIPIKA DELMENICO

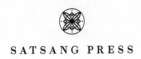

SATSANG PRESS

Copyright © 2018 by Dipika Delmenico

All rights reserved. No part of this book may be reproduced, stored in a retrieval system or transmitted, in any form or by any means, without the prior written consent of the publisher.

ISBN 978-0-64843-900-4 (paperback)
ISBN 978-0-64843-901-1 (ebook)

This book is not intended as a substitute for the medical advice of physicians. The reader should regularly consult a physician in matters relating to his/her health and particularly with respect to any symptoms that may require diagnosis or medical attention.

Produced by Page Two Books
www.pagetwobooks.com

Cover design by Prateeba Perumal
Interior design by Nayeli Jimenez
Editing by Kendra Ward
Proofreading by Alison Strobel

18 19 20 21 22   5 4 3 2 1

www.dipikadelmenico.com

I offer infinite love and eternal gratitude to the benevolent Grace of my Guru.
I offer infinite acknowledgment of my teachers.
I offer infinite gratitude to my teachers.
I offer infinite gratitude to my ancestral lineage of mothers.
I offer infinite gratitude to my daughters.

To beloved Ma Gaṅgā, my salutations. To you, I bow. To you, I offer all. Jai Ma.

To Lord Dhanvantari, salutations and gratitude for the gift of Ayurveda to humanity.

Saha Nā Vavatu Saha Nau Bhunaktu
Saha Vīryaṁ Karavāvahai
Tejasvināvadhītamastu Mā Vidviṣāvahai

(Together, may we learn from each other, protect, nourish, have strength to study and let it be without dislike or hostility)

I invite you to give gratitude and reverence to the archetypal mother, to the great feminine essence, to your ancestral lineage of mothers:

Those who have forged a path through love, courage, wisdom, compassion, and benevolent grace.
Those who have prayed and made sacrifices for you.
For the stories of women, the stories of your ancestral women, the songs.

To every woman, I offer this book as a gesture of my respect and gratitude for you.

Contents

· · · · · · · · · · · · ·

Introduction

. . . .

Revere woman. She is sublime.
Woman is called the mother of all.
She is supremely beloved.
Look on her with reverence.
SWAMI MUKTANANDA

THE GREAT FEMININE essence in each living being on the planet is calling to be healed right now, more than at any other time. As the ultimate keeper of Source, which is the infinite possibility to create life, women have a sacred duty to be connected to this feminine aspect of all life.

By exploring the ancient healing wisdom of Ayurveda and living life processes, you can embody this great feminine essence, your radiance as a woman. There are great mysteries known to you as a woman, and these mysteries are calling to be remembered.

In essence, you are already whole and complete. You have simply forgotten aspects of your true nature as a woman. This book is a tool to support your remembrance. As a wise woman shared with me, to remember (or "re-member") is to put all aspects of ourselves, even those we've forgotten, back together. When we remember, we realign.

A particular kind of awakening occurs within when you are brushed by truth. This truth has a certain kind of light and I am called to share this light with every woman, for we are truly all sisters, holding hands and moving to the ultimate heartbeat of the great mother.

It is my wish that this book empowers you to embody your radiance and potential as the magnificent woman you are.

Why This Book?

In a world with a dwindling capacity to imagine, wonder, focus, and feel, and even a diminishing inclination to read books, I am called to write one! I see myself as a messenger, an instrument of the divine wisdom of truth, meaning, and healing. I am a messenger of the sound of life, the resounding sound of the great feminine in you, in me, in each of us on this planet.

I am not separate from the air that moves in and out of my lungs, and the wind that moves the leaves on the trees. I am not separate from the water that nourishes and moistens the cells of my being and that provides a dwelling for the fishes, platypuses, whales, dolphins, sharks, and friends of the oceans, lakes, and rivers. Nor am I separate from the earth that gives my form stability to stand firm until ready to dissolve. I am not separate from the fire that forges the energy of my being and spark of light in my core. And I am not separate from the space that allows me to explore, feel, need, learn, teach, rest, grow, and love. I am eternally grateful to live in an environment where the forces and beauty of nature command me to go within myself and listen to the pulsating throb of my womanhood.

I am not separate from you.

The ancient keepers of wisdom are my friends, mentors, guardians, protectors, guides. They care for me, so I may dutifully share with others. To the record keepers of all life, I offer my infinite gratitude and a garland of love.

May this book be received in the fullness of silence. May it be lived in the fullness of silence. May it be lived through the great resounding feminine in you. You are vital: only your being can bring a unique sound to this planet. You are so precious. Although the great feminine can be seen and felt by the eyes and impulses of your heart, your intuition and all your senses, it is qualitative. It is resonant and possesses a particular sound, unique to each human being and woman—unique to you.

As a daughter, a "custodian" of all daughters, a mother, an auntie, a sister, I am compelled to be all I can possibly be so that my fellow woman can be all that she can be. I strive to be well in myself so that others can be well in themselves.

I invite you to reflect on your intention for reading this book, and what you hope to gain.

I

Ayurveda and the Sacred Feminine

CHAPTER 1

The Sound of Your Great Feminine

· · · · · · · · · · · ·

THE VEDAS SAY all righteousness, all wealth, abundance, and all of creation depend upon woman.

Dharmārthau Strīṣu Lakṣmīścha Strīṣu Lokāḥ Pratiṣṭhitāḥ

The great feminine is an energy inherent in each of us that has the potential for infinite possibilities. It is a source of mighty power. Although soft and nourishing, it is also formidable in capacity and capability. Women, as the archetypal expression of this feminine energy, are called to embody this source of womanhood. As the manifestation of the original mother, you as a woman must cultivate your intimate establishment with the great feminine.

All human beings can live to our fullest potential when we have a solid relationship with, understanding of, and connection to this aspect of ourselves.

Within each of us is a resonance, a reverberating sound that pulsates with life force and love. This throb pulsates with vitality and is like a beacon of our humanness.

For women, this is the sound of our womanhood. Call it ancient, wild, truth, source, the great feminine, it is *cit śakti*—the pulsating throb and play of consciousness. It is kuṇḍalinī śakti, the divine primordial energy of the universe. It is real. It is you. The more you connect with and live in intimacy with this throb, the more enlivened and aligned you are in your power.

My dearest woman, you cannot recognize or deeply understand this essence in another until you have heard and experienced this sound in yourself. You may have an idea of it, but until you experience the sound of this feminine energy in its deep penetration, it will remain conceptual. I urge you to listen with your heart to this resounding sound, for it is also the sound of nature, the sound of Mother Earth.

This is the sound of your vitality, the sound of your effulgence, the sound of your radiance.

When kuṇḍalinī awakes, the eyes are filled with light,
Fragrance rises, nectar bathes the tongue,
ecstasy plays in the heart.
Citti is Lakṣmi,
She is Sarasvāti and Kali.
The cosmos is pervaded by Her.
Dear woman, the citti without is kuṇḍalinī within.
SWAMI MUKTANANDA

When I play my tānpūrā out of tune, I do not experience the full, clear resonance I am seeking. It's all right, but it's not refined or pure. When I sing without warming up my voice, it is clunky and dense. When I speak or act without tuning myself via inner reflection or meditation, these words and actions, too, can be somewhat coarse.

We tune ourselves every day in order to stay connected to this divine resonance of our own essence. This is the music of our life, our cosmic symphony sounding its absolute best. What a performance, indeed. Instruments do not stay in tune without our intention, attention, and care.

So what is the point of this tuning and care in relation to you as a divine human being? You are an instrument of God. The divine universal spirit is played through you. Honor the entire symphony by staying in tune, dear woman.

There is so much coming at you in modern life, each and every day. Emails. Advertisements. Intellectual property. Fear-based campaigns. Sell, sell, sell. Market, market, market. Automate. There's a constant loud, busy drone of all of these messages. The constant hum of it can be too much. How do you discern what is beneficial among all this relentless information?

Our calendars can be full or overbooked, even overlooked. I use alarms for reminders and prompts. We live in a world of apps. There are even apps for going to bed or breathing. Really? Have we forgotten when and how to put ourselves to bed, how to take a breath, how to be mindful? Surely this way of living can become disempowering and can even take away from your very autonomy as a woman. I urge you to contemplate where you are going, and to tenderly use the wise and all-knowing supports of nature to help you find your pathway.

A bridge links you between this earthly realm and the spirit world. At times the veils that obscure this bridge and your remembrance of it and its purpose are forgotten. At other times you may use this bridge as a regular thoroughfare, traveling to-and-fro, giving and receiving. Just as you are nourished by the spirit world, the spirit world is nourished by you.

Shamans cross this bridge. Mystics know it. Children know it. Initiates since time immemorial know it. This bridge is there for each of us, and it belongs to each of us.

It could well be that the very foundations and materials that compose this bridge are of vibration. Everything in the universe is composed of sound, including yourself. To really thrive and make sense of the task of being human, I believe we must get familiar with how to cross this bridge.

You obtained your body by God's grace.
It is a precious gift and deserves right use.
Use it for meditation.
You will drink the nectar of immortality.
There is one who lives in the body,
Who pervades it and knows it through and through.
Dear woman, that inner knower is your nature.
SWAMI MUKTANANDA

The great feminine essence is calling to be healed in each of us, now more than at any other time on the planet. By exploring living life processes and the ancient healing wisdom of Ayurveda, we merge with this great feminine essence.

Pūrṇamadaḥ Pūrṇamidam
Pūrṇāt Pūrṇamudacyate
Pūrṇasya Pūrṇamādāya
Pūrṇamevā Vaśiṣyate

This is perfect
That is perfect
If you take the perfect away from the perfect
Only the perfect remains.

My dear ones, you are whole and complete in essence. This book will remind you of this fact: Wholeness is your very nature, though you have forgotten it. We all forget, and my wish is for you to remember.

CHAPTER 2

Ayurveda, a Gift
to Humanity

· · · · · · · · · · · · ·

BEFORE SOUND WAS silence, and this harmonious silence was composed of energy, vibration, consciousness, and light.

Over five thousand years ago, humankind suffered from many kinds of diseases. In essence, the condition of spirit was manifesting itself as a spectrum of *disease*: ailments of the physical body, the mind, the emotions, and even the soul.

A group of sages went to Lord Indra, the King of Gods, asking for a solution. The sages practiced this science known as "Ayurveda," *ayu* meaning life and *veda* meaning knowledge. Lord Indra passed the knowledge containing such solutions to Lord Dhanvantari. In their compassion for humankind, the great enlightened rishis gifted Ayurveda to humanity, giving them the means to heal themselves from illnesses through the ability to remember one's nature when one deviated away from nature herself. These rishis could see it was difficult to navigate life as a woman, to experience and make meaning of our very womanhood. Ayurveda was given as a tool for understanding our nature so that all beings could live aligned with heart, truth, and soul purpose.

These rishis lived in the fullness of silence, and from silence they uttered the sounds of the letters of Sanskrit, the science and knowledge of life. Sanskrit is the language of the Gods. Its very letters embody the resonance and vibrations of the entire cosmos. Ayurveda as we know it was recorded in the ancient scriptural texts, the Vedas. The classical Ayurvedic treatises, *Caraka Saṁhitā* and *Suśruta Saṁhitā*, were recorded in 4000 BCE.

Ayurveda is a philosophy for living a balanced life. This philosophy works in any era or country, for all groups of people. Ayurveda is composed of the source from which you are manifested and to which you return. People are born into all manner of circumstances. We have our own inherent constitutions, which bring strengths and weaknesses. Our task is to overcome, grow, and love within these constitutions. We begin by loving what we have. The Ayurvedic woman loves herself for the miracle she is.

There is a fundamental need to understand, to assimilate, and to have meaning. The striving to experience this connection is yoga, meaning "union," between body and mind and spirit. The tools with which to have this experience are Ayurveda.

Ayurveda and Modern Life

Although this rich, insightful, and practical philosophy has been around for thousands of years, Ayurveda is as practical today as when first imparted to us. In fact, as long as human beings live on this planet, Ayurveda will have no use-by date: It will always have relevance for our lives.

Life is loud, crowded, noisy, and hot. We are heating up and hardening. Ayurveda gives us the tools to cool and pacify ourselves, to remain soft and malleable. We simply have to follow these principles and use these tools to see how effective they really are. Using

Ayurveda will support you to navigate your life in a meaningful and enlightened way.

Although our contemporary issues may seem more complicated than those of our ancestors, we still face the same emotions, feelings, and inward challenges. Heart is heart, emotion is emotion, pain is pain, suffering is suffering, and need is need. There is no emotion, need, or pain new to us. Ayurveda gives us the means to balance, strengthen, and nourish this aspect of ourselves.

Ayurveda is a path of moderation. Its key is to balance and align in such a way that you can feel, think, and see clearly, from a place of equilibrium. A moderate way of living, closely to nature, allows you to fully enjoy this experience of life and stay well. It is really only when you fall out of rhythm and balance within your own nature that it becomes necessary to abstain from certain things, in order to come back to center again.

Only you can make the time to create health-promoting habits for yourself. They do not have to be huge. Keep it small. Keep it simple. Make it part of your daily schedule and you will feel the benefits in all aspects of your life. This way of living works because it is authentic and supports you the way that nature intended.

These principles help you to live meaningfully and purposefully, in a way that contributes and uplifts not only you, but others and our very planet.

The Six Tools of Ayurveda

Ayurveda is a complete, holistic life science. It is a healing system that does not treat the symptoms of an illness; instead, it focuses on addressing the root cause of the ailment.

Symptoms are manifestations of a deeper imbalance within the body or the mind. Pain tells us something is wrong, but if all we do is take a pain reliever, the pain will return. Ayurveda teaches us to look at the underlying cause of the symptoms and work to cure it.

Once you resolve the root cause of an imbalance, the symptoms will disappear naturally.

There are six tools of Ayurveda:

1. **Diet:** The Ayurvedic diet is focused on the six tastes: sweet, salty, sour, pungent, bitter, and astringent.

2. **Lifestyle:** By living a balanced life, your body is better able to resist and fight off illness and disease.

3. **Herbal Remedies:** As all life is composed of five elements—earth, air, fire, water, and ether (meaning space)—herbal remedies made of these elements can be used therapeutically to support healing in all aspects of your body and mind.

4. **Home Remedies:** The life science of Ayurveda contains an abundance of home remedies that, if used properly, can help address your underlying illness. These home remedies are effective in acute and chronic situations.

5. **Panchakarma:** This is a deep cleansing and rejuvenating program for the mind, body, and soul.

6. **Marma:** This is a specialized massage technique that focuses on the vital energy points of the body. By gently manipulating these points, a skilled practitioner can help restore natural balance to their patient's body and being. Marma therapy is used for physical, emotional, and mental health conditions.

The Basics of Ayurvedic Philosophy

All matter consists of five basic elements. Human beings, animals, and plants are all microcosms within nature and hence each of the five elements is within each individual. A balance of these five elements is responsible for all life force on the planet:

1. **Earth:** This element represents solidity, nourishment, and steadiness. It is our bones and muscles.

2. **Water:** This element represents moisture, fluidity, and nourishment. It is our blood and plasma.

3. **Fire:** This element represents transformation, metabolism, and heat. It is our hormones, enzymes, digestive juices, and other natural processes.

4. **Air:** This element is transportation and motion. It is our nerve impulses and all movement of the body.

5. **Ether (space):** This element is emptiness. It is found in our hollow organs, such as our gastrointestinal tract and circulatory system.

By identifying where the underlying imbalance lies, and within which element, Ayurveda can help you treat the fundamental issues that are affecting your life.

The five basic elements present as three attributes called *dośas*. The dośas, or biological humors, are responsible for human existence. They are *vata*, *pitta*, and *kapha*:

1. **Vata:** This attribute is composed of ether and air. It is the principle of movement and motion in the body and mind.

2. **Pitta:** This attribute is fire. It is the principle of energy, the transformation of each organism.

3. **Kapha:** This attribute is composed of water and earth. It is the principle of structure and cohesion. It stabilizes, lubricates, and maintains.

Each of the dośas is formed with the characteristics of the corresponding element and is a catalyst for several functions within the body, such as digestion, respiration, elimination, formation, and growth. You cannot see dośas, yet their presence is felt. They pervade the body, constantly working in each cell. When they are in balance, the doṣas preserve the rhythm and balance of organisms. An imbalance of doṣas creates disease.

The doṣas constantly work in each cell of the body. They concentrate in those tissues where they are particularly needed:

- Vata is particularly active in the nervous system, circulatory system and heart, large intestine, bones, lungs, pelvis, and ears.

- Pitta concentrates in the liver, spleen, small intestine, endocrine glands, skin, eyes, blood, and sweat.

- Kapha is most concentrated in the joints, upper respiratory system, stomach, lymph, thorax and fat.

Every person is born with a particular constitution, your individual blueprint from conception. In Ayurveda this is your prakṛti. Balance happens when each doṣa is in alignment. Of course, we are fluid beings constantly in motion, not fixed or static. Our doṣas constantly seek a state of harmony. That means they are adjusting themselves, always fine-tuning. For example, if there is too little pitta, it will strive to increase. If there is too much, or if pitta is aggravated, it will strive to be pacified. Each person is born with certain doṣas in dominance. Depending on diet, lifestyle, environmental, climatic, and other factors, certain doṣas increase or decrease. When the doṣas are out of balance, we lose equilibrium of mental, emotional, and physical health. This imbalance is called vikṛti. This is your body's current condition.

It's been my experience over decades of clinical practice that people are so eager to know what their constitution is. "What is my doṣa?" is the commonly asked question. Simply put, people wish to understand themselves in order to find meaning. Although it may be helpful to know your doṣa, in order to navigate gracefully through life, it's really helpful to know your vikṛti—that is, what is happening for you right now? What dynamic forces are currently at play?

Attributes of the Dośas

As forces, the dośas have particular attributes, qualities, and energetics. Once you have a sense of these qualities, then you can feel into them, becoming familiar with them in yourself and in all living things. This allows you to know yourself and create vitality, meaning, and wellness. You can understand the nature of things through knowing the qualities of these governing forces.

QUALITIES

VATA	PITTA	KAPHA
Dry	Oily	Oily
Cold	Hot	Cold
Light	Light	Heavy
Irregular	Intense	Stable
Mobile	Fluid	Viscous
Erratic	Malodorous	Dense
Rough	Liquid	Smooth

ENERGY OF THE DOŚAS

Each of the dośas lend themselves to particular characteristics and ways of using energy:

- Vata people tend to spend energy freely and wastefully. This energetic nature exerts a cold, dry, irregular influence on a biological system. Hence this energy often comes in bursts and is short-lived. Vata qualities encourage energy to be expended as soon as it enters an organism. It's like an all-or-nothing expression. Vata, although it may fluctuate between dilation and constriction, encourages restriction.

- Pitta people possess driving energy that produces a hot, oily, intense, and irritable effect. The pitta humor must maintain a high level of reactivity to use its energy effectively. This is why pitta people can burn out or even overcook. Pitta creates a dilation of channels.

- Kapha people have slow, steady energy. It is a potential energy that lends a predisposition to save and store well. Kapha promotes congestion.

CONSTITUTIONAL CHARACTERISTICS

Vata is the subtle energy that governs breathing, blinking, movements, nerve impulses, and the pulse. It also governs feelings and emotions.

Vata people do things quickly. They also change quickly—there is an irregularity to vata. They can have great energy some days, with strong digestion, and have a good sleep. The next they can feel flat, with poor digestion or appetite, and have an erratic, light sleep. Elimination can swing from loose bowels to constipation, with a tendency for the latter. Energy typically comes in spurts. The physical body and mind tend toward restlessness. Much energy is used on things that they become easily addicted to. The body tends to be lean, dry, rough, and cold. The mind is imaginative. Often insecure and ungrounded, vata emotions may constantly waver. The unbalanced emotion tends to be fear or anxiety. Vata people are changeable.

Pitta is the heat energy of the body. It governs digestion, absorption, assimilation, nutrition, metabolism, temperature, complexion, eye luster, intelligence, and understanding. Pitta triggers anger, hate, jealousy, irritability.

Pitta people are physically and mentally efficient and effective, which can make them critical of themselves and others. They tend to dislike heat unless addicted to the stimulation of it. Generally, their warm, soft, freckly, or pimply skin does not react well to sun or heat. Of strong mind, they often try to impose this will upon others. Pitta types have the best digestion, with a strong appetite. They can be grumpy or irritable if they skip a meal or feel hungry. They can be competitive and impatient with those not learning something as fast as they do. They can be easily one-pointed in their focus, in order to be successful with it. They are sharp and intelligent. The natural heat of pitta creates courage when well harnessed and disciplined; otherwise, the predominant emotion can be anger. Most pitta disease is created by physical and mental heat. The physical body tends to be moderate, warm, and lustrous in complexion. Pitta people represent intensity.

Kapha gives the materials for our physical structure. It is responsible for biological strength and the natural resistance of the body. It lubricates joints, moisturizes skin, heals wounds, fills spaces in the body, and gives vigor and stability. It is responsible for emotions of greed and attachment. It creates calmness, love, forgiveness.

Kapha people, who like to live slow and relaxed, tend to be solidly built. They gain weight easily and lose it with difficulty unless exercising regularly. They tend to have well-nourished bodies and sleep long and deeply. They may learn more slowly, but they have good memory and rarely forget. They can be prone to congestive complaints. Possessing the attributes of earth, they are grounded and steady. They possess great stamina and can easily skip meals without discomfort. They can be complacent and adverse to change when it's needed.

Symptom Evaluation

Imbalanced or aggravated dośas, unless addressed, can cause symptoms. Sometimes they pathologize in combination with *aam*. Aam is a metabolic sludge composed of a partially digested substance that putrefies and blocks, becoming poisonous to our physiology and all aspects of our being. Aam will interfere with free movement and activity of the dośas.

A general rule about symptoms offers insight into the primary nature of dośa imbalances:

- **Vata = pain:** There is no pain without vata involvement (for example, colic-type pain is vata pain).

- **Pitta = inflammation:** There is no inflammation without pitta (for example, ulcers or sunburns are pitta pain).

- **Kapha = pus:** There is no pus formation without kapha (for example, congested, stuffed nose is kapha pain).

The following are common vata symptoms:
- tachycardia
- heart palpitations
- diarrhea (increased movement)
- cramps, numbness (decreased movement)
- convulsions, tremors (distorted movement)
- prolapses
- cracked skin (separation of tissue from one another)

The following are common pitta symptoms:
- indigestion
- heartburn
- burning diarrhea
- fever
- burning sensations
- inflammations
- ulcerations
- blood and bleeding disorders
- rashes
- jaundice
- anemia

The following are common kapha symptoms:
- excessive mucus
- respiratory congestion

- pallor
- sluggishness
- heaviness of body (and limbs)
- itching

Dhātus

There are seven different types of bodily tissues, or *dhātus*. They vary in quality from the grossest to the subtlest. It's important to have some understanding of these dhātus because they are created by the kind of foods we eat, and they are responsible for the most refined residual energy you possess. This energy is your *ojas*, your vital life energy.

According to Ayurveda, the divine creator places a drop of ojas in the center of each human's heart and we are given the task of nourishing this drop through our life. Once depleted and gone, there is no more life.

Here is a table of the seven types of bodily tissues, their qualities and functions. Although dhātus are physical tissues, each dhātu has a qualitative influence and effect on emotions and the mind.

THE SEVEN DHĀTUS

DHĀTU	TISSUE	EMOTIONAL/ MENTAL QUALITATIVE EFFECT	FUNCTIONS
rasa	plasma and lymph	feeling of enough, satisfaction, contentment	Nourishes all the tissues of the body. Gives juiciness to one's being. Helps elimination and quenches mental thirst. Nourishes *rakta dhātu*.
rakta	blood	conscious intelligence	Carrier and supplier of vital life energies, including *prāṇa* (breath), and vehicle for consciousness. Gives luster and glow to skin. Nourishes *māmsa dhātu*.

DHĀTU	TISSUE	EMOTIONAL/ MENTAL QUALITATIVE EFFECT	FUNCTIONS
māmsa	muscle	courage, stability, steadfastness, patience	Integrity and strength of the body's muscle tissue. Nourishes *medha dhātu*.
medha	fat (adipose)	softness, soothing, generosity	Gives lubrication to all the body tissues. Generates sweat. Nourishes *asthi dhātu*.
asthi	bone	emotional and mental resilience and robustness	Nourishes bone tissue to give proper strength and structure of the body. Nourishes *majja dhātu*.
majja	nerve and marrow	refined resonance	Gives strength and intelligence to space occupied in the lumen by nerve activity. Nourishes *śukra dhātu*.
śukra	reproductive	courage, vitality, love, joy	Gives quality and function of reproductive tissues and organs. Imparts mental strength.

THE LIVING LIFE PROCESSES

Dr. Rudolf Steiner, an Austrian philosopher, introduced the principles of seven life processes in *Course for Young Doctors*, a series of lectures to medical doctors (1909, 1916). This vast subject of esoteric science encompasses all of life and living forces. Just as the dośas in Ayurvedic philosophy are not something that can actually be seen, so, too, are these living forces of life processes. The terms Dr. Steiner used for these are:

- breathing
- warming
- nourishing
- secreting
- maintaining
- growing
- regenerating (reproducing)

These seven life processes are part of the basic understanding of the human being through the lens of anthroposophy and anthroposophical medicine. This approach to understanding and healing a human is so rich, curative, and completely holistic. These principles and themes are woven into my understanding of what constitutes woman in all her mystery, on all levels and aspects of her seasons and being, and thus they form a living part of this book.

In his 2006 book A Living Physiology, Dr. Karl König, medical doctor and founder of the Camphill Movement, elaborates on the seven life processes so succinctly and eloquently. These are:

- **Breathing:** In breathing, we communicate with the world. Breathing is essentially what we call "rhythm," the coming and going that connects us like an umbilical cord to the world.

- **Warming:** What has been inhaled becomes permeated by warmth, which gives inner form to the inhalation of breath from the outside world.

- **Nourishment:** The warmth in permeated form takes in nourishment.

König notes that these three living processes, as soon as they are established, create a response from within, which is the secreting. Working with the breathing, warming, and nourishment, the secretion transforms what has been taken in. It maintains and makes its own. From here there can be growth, which leads to regeneration.

These "ladder-like" living processes possess a sevenfold quality (just like the seven levels of tissues, or seven major energy centers, cakras). They can be looked at like an overarching archetypal image of living processes in us.

II

General Cycles

CHAPTER 3

Digestion for Life

· · · · · · · · · · · ·

TO ESTABLISH YOUR digestion for life, it's necessary to have some understanding of your great feminine essence—the seed sound of your womanhood.

Digestion is the seat of good health. Five thousand years ago, Ayurveda was onto it and said it's the key to your longevity and good vitality. Simple in principle, it means keeping your gut function strong and clean. Keep your bodily tissue clean. Keep the tissues of the mental channels clean. Ayurveda completely, holistically understands the energy and nature of digestion.

What, then, is the fire of digestion? Warmth is necessary for any digestive process to occur. This warmth is what cooks, transforms, and transmutes anything and everything we are to digest.

Our *agni* is our digestive fire. We not only have to digest everything we ingest as food, we also must digest what we ingest environmentally (including all chemicals and pollutants, pollens, dusts, fumes, and perfumes).

When we ingest any kind of food, we have to overcome its nature, which is inherently foreign to our body. You could say that food is a poison and our task is to overcome—to digest and destruct it. To be able to digest is to be able to break down and prevail.

Of paramount significance is that we must also digest every single life experience and impression we have from the moment we are born. Yes, this is a mammoth and ongoing task. It means digesting all the feelings of the heart and experiences of the mind. It means being able to digest what is experienced in the mental channels. Thus it is necessary to have the right kind of warmth in the organism. Having the right digestive fire is vital to the innate capacity to process your experience of life.

You could say that the right understanding gives the right warmth and the right warmth equates to the right understanding. And these two, together, give us integrity. This is a mighty big job, and it's constant.

Nature in her benevolent grace has the capacity to do this job effectively and efficiently so that you can remain vital and thrive. However, like anything in nature, it is necessary to follow a prescribed formula in order to experience this strong digestion. In this book, I share these alchemical digestive formulas.

If you are unable to digest certain foods, if you have sensitivity, allergic reactions, discomfort of any kind or intolerance to certain foods, then your digestive function needs to be strengthened. You will show negative responses and reactions, inflammatory responses, to more and more foods unless you strengthen and improve your digestion.

The long-term solution is not to remove more and more foods from your diet. To remove foods from your diet ultimately contracts your life and narrows your world. You are a social being. Your role is to engage, interact, share, give, and receive with other people. Hence, the long-term solution for sensitivities and allergies is to bolster and manage your ability to digest. You do this by bolstering your fire of digestion, thereby nourishing and cultivating the warmth of the digestive organism.

When speaking of allergic reactions, this does not include extreme, life-threatening allergic reactions, like anaphylaxis. If you have an extreme allergy to, say, seafood, peanuts, even mangoes, you must carry emergency medication to manage yourself. Although it is still most beneficial to keep digestion optimal and as strong as can be, to manage inflammation and reactivity, certain foods will always be best avoided in this instance. However, the same principle applies: Continuously tend to and manage your digestive capacity.

Your fire of digestion needs regular attention. You, as keeper of the fire, must stoke it. Not too much, nor too little. The fire needs to be very rhythmic and constant. It is always necessary to foster the right warmth of the organism.

Even with autoimmune diseases, such as celiac disease, which are becoming more common, digestion is key to stabilizing and creating good immune stability, function, and vitality. A celiac who has a gluten intolerance will never be able to eat and tolerate gluten without an inflammatory response. However, for a person with celiac disease, the key to their good health is to keep the digestive fire strong so that they can digest the foods they can tolerate.

Josie is forty-eight years old. She has celiac disease. When I first saw her in her late thirties she was suffering greatly. Her digestion was so compromised that she had a great aversion to cooking food for herself. She was eating takeaway and fried food and drinking carbonated caffeinated drinks. She was frustrated, depressed, overwhelmed, and had a low sense of worth. She spent much time loathing herself.

We worked together gently and diligently with Ayurvedic herbs, which are gentle formulations, and home remedies. The herbal remedies worked on all levels of digestion: physical gut digestion, emotional digestion, and mental digestion. We worked to bring down the inflammation. There was much inflammation in not only the gut but the mental channels, meaning there was an aggravation and excess of metabolic heat, which fed her self-loathing and aversion to self-care. The home remedies were simple, including beginning Josie's day with a teaspoon of ghee in hot water before breakfast. Over time, Josie's mood stabilized. She no longer lived with a constant sense of self-loathing and overwhelm. She began to feel empowered, with greater appetite and capacity to prepare food for herself. Her physical energy improved and her quality of sleep became more refreshing. Josie now cleanses periodically to reduce inflammation and to work qualitatively with her mind. She will always avoid wheat in her diet but her digestive capacity is now so much stronger and her physical and mental channel tissue is cleaner. Josie is empowered, and her radiance is a joy to experience.

The body is essentially about communication—flow—through a wild and intricate system of channels, with vessels of all shapes and sizes from the grossest to the subtlest and finest. All these channels are dependent on process and flow. The functioning and thriving of the body are dependent on this process and flow. It dictates the effectiveness of the communication.

Blockages in channels are a major cause of all kinds of health problems, creating disease. When there's blockage, there is lack of ease and harmony. It means movement is obstructed. Effective communication is not possible and processes are not efficient. When this occurs, flow needs to be reinstated, unimpeded. Problems with all aspects of your being, including mental, emotional, physical, and soul life, can be experienced when there are blockages in these channels because vitality is impacted.

The problems can manifest in multiple ways and can be experienced as poor concentration, lack of focus, dullness of mood, lack of enthusiasm, lack of tolerance, memory challenges, lack of refreshing sleep, arthritic aches and pains, respiratory complaints, digestive and gut complaints, dizziness, vertigo, balance, weight issues, atrophy, and low enthusiasm for life.

When you are working on digestion, you are working on removing blockages. Hence, we always focus on diet to balance the doṣas, or governing forces, and to bring them back to their normal path of movement. The focus is on removing blockages, improving circulation and metabolism. We thereby improve the quality of digestion and tissue in the body, our dhātus.

Practical Tools for Good Digestion for Life

According to Ayurveda, some simple fundamental principles can establish good digestion for life. One of these is moderation: not too much, not too little, not too frequently nor too infrequently. You can celebrate life with chocolate mud cake today for a birthday celebration, but that does not mean you have to eat it tomorrow, the day after, or every day. Typically, we are not masters of being moderate. When we discover something that we enjoy, we tend to overdo it and are immoderate in our consumption. Moderation means having the right understanding and good digestion.

Ayurveda encourages us to cook the majority of our food. Everything we ingest has to be converted into a nourishing substance that can be absorbed by the body. Food turns into fuel that ultimately nourishes our soul life. Along the way it gives us vitality so that we can be of service and do the tasks required of us in order to experience a good quality of our soul life. Unless we cook the food first, the gut has to cook it 100 percent with the warmth of our digestive fire, which can be a huge ongoing task to ask of our gut. Particularly with challenges and stressors, such as trauma, shock, grief, and times of crisis, our digestive energy is often dispersed elsewhere in the body. At these times our gut function is not as strong, as the energy is being directed to help us cope. In illness, digestive energy is directed to help the body overcome the illness, and as such digestion is compromised. Its focus at this time is to support our immunity. Just as with women's menstruation each month, the digestive energy goes to support the menstrual cycle's reproductive function. The channels are open at such times and it is important to eat lightly and not overeat during menstruation so as not to burden the tissue.

Raw food has more nutritional substance than cooked food, but the key is being able to utilize and take up this substance. Generally speaking, in Ayurveda we avoid too much raw food because it is cold and heavy on the gut. Even salad leaves! Although they look light and refreshing, they are, in fact, heavy to digest and can create a lot of gas and air in the body.

Fresh vegetable juices are an exception. When taken on an empty stomach, they are instantly assimilated as a nourishing substance. They are liquid gold and highly nutritious. They keep up our juiciness of being, our lymph and plasma, our rasa dhātu.

More cooked foods are particularly helpful as we age. When we age, the air and gases naturally increase in the tissues and body. But, with awareness, we can continuously pacify our vata internally and bring this dośa back to its normal path of movement. Cooked foods support this process to happen.

Eating your meals in a relaxed environment is important. Loud, stressful environments, at the desk, checking social media, computer balanced on your lap, and food in hand, do not meet that criteria! Chew food slowly; focus on your food; say a blessing for the food; have gratitude for the food.

It has always has been a challenge for me to eat slowly, and it's particularly tricky as a mother. Often the first meal of the day is eaten standing up while preparing school lunches and serving breakfast to my children. However, standing up and eating on the go are not ideal nor conducive for good digestion, just as it's not necessary to overeat by eating not only my own meal but food left on my children's plates.

You can bring the right element of agni into your eating environment by lighting a candle at your meal. This is such a rich ritual, for children especially. A candle snuffer ensures good recordkeeping for whose turn it is to put out the candle at the end of the meal.

Appendix B includes general Ayurvedic diet guidelines that address these principles and suggest food combinations for optimal digestion, digestive spices, and the like.

It generally takes three to four hours to fully digest a meal (it takes longer to digest heavy, rich meals with meat, fried foods, lots of dairy, or combinations of dairy and meat). This speed changes for people depending on their inherent constitution. Vata-dominant people thrive on eating smaller meals more frequently and even grazing between meals. Pitta-dominant people thrive on eating meals every four hours, and people with more kapha digest much slower and sometimes feel better when they miss a meal.

A healthy appetite means that three to four hours after your last meal you have a real hunger for more food. If you have an empty feeling your gut within two hours of eating a substantial meal, then your digestion needs attention. For example, when somebody has too much metabolic heat in the small intestine, there can be an "all gone" feeling, they can be weak in the body, and experience tiredness, a real fatigue. Nutrients are moving too quickly through the body and not assimilating well. This malnutrition of the tissues is not because somebody is not eating nutrient-dense food, but rather there is an assimilation glitch because of the excess metabolic heat.

Sometimes, an accumulation of sludge in the gut will mask the proper digestion and nourishment. You can feel hungry and, in fact, you are, but it's a false or faulty appetite because of this layer of mucosal-like sludge coating the intestinal wall and hence affecting absorption.

If you do not have a strong appetite at mealtime, it may be that you have been eating too much between meals or your digestion simply needs some support.

A great way to bolster digestion before meals is to sip on ginger tea, or even Amara bitters. It will recalibrate digestion so that the gut will wake up to what is has to do. Remember Amara bitters as a great remedy to always have on hand when traveling—the bitters help digestion when it's confused by new time zones, climatic conditions, and the like. It helps the body know it's not upside down and is able to take a meal in and digest it well.

Sipping on ginger tea after meals also aids digestion. Even sipping on hot water after a meal aids the digestive process, as well as keeping vata pacified.

It is encouraged not to drink too much water with meals because this essentially dilutes the digestive fire and juices. Also, digestion thrives by drinking water and liquids at room temperature. Ice-cold drinks straight from the fridge, ice in drinks, and carbonated drinks all dampen the digestive fire.

Digestion will weaken as you age and you naturally become drier. Soupy stew, like one-pot meals, help as they keep tissue pacified and nourished. Skin become thinner as you age. You can nourish the skin by regularly massaging yourself with warm oil, and ingesting oils and nourishing foods.

Eating meals at regular times is key for supporting digestion. When the sun is at its highest, your digestion is at its strongest. This means that you can eat your biggest meal most effortlessly at this time of day. Although this does not fit easily with our modern lives, you will thrive by eating something of considerable nourishment and sustenance at your midday meal. It is not a meal to be skipped. A handful of crackers and dip or carrot sticks will not cut it, nor will a bowl of lettuce or salad leaves.

Even though it is important for a family to eat a meal together, for the nourishment, ritual, and rhythm of family life, and this is often an evening meal, be mindful of still having considerable nourishment with the noon meal. I encourage you to have a smaller portion at evening meals to support optimum digestion.

Your good digestion creates a healthy flow between the metabolic organs, the gut, and all the mental-channels and nerve sense system, your emotions, your heart, your lungs, your prāṇa (breath). All metabolic processes must pass through the great rhythmic organs and balancing regulators of digestion.

The key is to be in touch with your feelings and needs and to nourish this rhythmic regulator for your well-being and vitality. The regulator of digestion is the starting point of any health issue as well as your ongoing wellness, vitality, and longevity. Good digestion equals good immunity. Good immune integrity means emotional intelligence and ojas, your vitality. So, when we increase our agni, our digestive fire, our metabolic function is improved. Our metabolism is linked with the health of tissues and digestive fires that govern each level of tissue in the body.

When we work with digestion, we address the root of problems, and symptoms disappear. The governing forces, the doṣas, become pacified and function more efficiently. This means you have more enthusiasm, life energy, efficient processes and optimal flow, and better communication.

When you improve digestion, respiration works more efficiently; you are more connected to the feelings of the heart; you can listen more clearly to your inner guidance. You eliminate more efficiently, and you feel lighter in being. Your resonance and vibration become lighter. It's a beautiful dance.

Bolster Digestion of Life Experiences

When you make time to nourish your digestion, creating daily space for contemplation, inner reflection, and meditation, you make a tonic that can digest and transmute all your impressions and experiences. This tonic supports your optimum digestion and vice versa. It creates a healthy flow between the metabolic organs, the gut, the nervous system and the mental channels because such activity nourishes your emotional life. It nourishes your heart, your inhalation and exhalation.

In this lemniscate, the top curve is your nerve sense system, where nerve sensory function is dominant. The lower curve is where all your organs of metabolism are housed, your organs of will. And in the center lie the great regulating organs of equilibrium, your rhythmic system. These organs are your heart and lungs. It is in

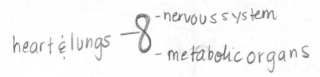

this rhythmic region that all your feelings and needs, not only as a woman but as a human, are housed. For good digestion of life, a flow of communication and process must remain effective, clear, and in rhythmic resonance between the upper and lower curves of nerve sensory function and metabolic function via your feeling heart, via the very capacity to be breathed by life and to breathe life.

The key to digestion here is in the connection to your heart, which keeps the very sound of the nerve sense activity integrated with the metabolic activity and vice versa. Circulating, reverberating and in a sense, homogenizing.

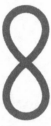

Digestion is always a starting point with any health issue.

Good digestion = immune integrity = emotional intelligence = ojas, wellness, vitality, longevity.

CHAPTER 4

Warmth

. . . .

WARMTH IS VITAL for the health of each organism. In its capacity to perform and ability to regulate heat, the warmth organization of the human body is extraordinary. For your wellness and health, the right kind of warmth is required by each organism in your very being.

An inner warmth is generated as part of a digestive process, maintained by the subcutaneous fat tissue in the body. This warmth is self-generated in perception and relationship to others and the environment. There is also a warmth process that is not as noticeable as body heat. This kind of warmth is a physical expression of inner light, which is also generated within each organism.

When proteins are broken down and digested in the blood, they are experienced as inner warmth. Likewise, the nervous system's activity is experienced as an inner light. This light is not the nerves themselves; it is the activity of the nerves.

We do not nourish ourselves by food alone, eaten in the right quantity and quality; we nourish ourselves when our inner processes are working in the right way. This is the right kind of warmth required by the body to keep vitality robust.

Cultivating your inner soul life generates and supports the right kind of warmth. Inner reflection and attention are necessary to thrive. If the warmth of inner movement and activity is not produced in the right way, you cannot react properly, leading to a lack of harmony or disease. Illness is an expression of the condition of your inner life, of your spirit. You could say it's a disturbance of the warmth organism.

CHAPTER 5

Cycles and Rhythms

. . . .

AS A WOMAN, you share a sacred rhythm with all other women. Your cyclic nature and the rhythms that influence all aspects of your health also give you understanding of yourself and life. This chapter explores the link between nature's cycles, innate rhythms, healthy hormones, and metabolic processes as the crucial key to your vitality.

Breath flows in, breath flows out,
Traveling always the curving path of the Goddess.
Breath flows spontaneously of its own will.
Thus all breathing beings
Continually give reverence to Her.
Be conscious of this unconscious prayer,
For She is the most holy place of pilgrimage.
She wishes for you to enter this temple,
Where each breath is adoration
Of the infinite for the incarnate form.
...The flowers, the incense,

Grain, spices, and honey
Offered in ritual
Are made out of the same divine stuff as you.
Who then is worshipped?
INSIGHT VERSE 154, *THE RADIANCE SUTRAS*

We live in a world of rhythms. Rhythms, patterns, and cycles within themselves, with varying circles of influence, all affected by one another, resonating, pulsating, vibrating.

There are seasonal rhythms, monthly rhythms, daily rhythms, circadian rhythms, digestive rhythms, metabolic rhythms.

When we sit with nature and watch her, we are sitting in and observing rhythms. There is regularity and routine to each of these. There are patterns, mathematics, sacred geometry. You are a custodian of the rhythm of life force.

Many years ago, while I was living in a yoga ashram in India, a fellow ashramite told me that I was like the reluctant yogi. I resisted the structure and discipline of the daily schedule. This was so true. I drew an image of myself with arms crossed and teeth clenched, resisting the very thing I knew and came to love and cherish so dearly: the daily rhythm. The discipline and regularity of the daily schedule gave me steadfast wellness and freedom. I thrived in all aspects of myself when I let go of resistance and embraced this daily rhythm.

This realization is something I have come to understand and respect enormously. When I am floundering or feeling unhinged, I come back to this daily rhythm like a life jacket keeping me buoyant in turbulent waters. I have observed that people who possess the great virtue of contentment adhere to a daily rhythm in their life.

We all thrive in daily rhythm. Our children thrive in it. All we have to do is establish it! Our children will simply follow by imitation. It's what they do. A child's thriving with daily routine and rhythms illustrates how we all thrive when we observe nature's patterns.

Cultivating healthy daily routines gives great benefit to your well-being. The mind is nurtured, faith and self-confidence build, focus and mind power grow, steady reserves of mental stamina and energy to experience positiveness throughout the day are developed. Daily rhythm imparts equanimity.

If a vessel has a hole in it, then water will constantly leak out and cannot be fully shaped and held by that vessel. The structure of daily rhythm plugs the holes and stops the leakage of our precious life force in ways that do not serve us. In this way, daily rhythm grounds, anchors, and harnesses our vitality.

Some folk are born with a steady daily rhythm; some folk inherently embody it. Some are raised to revere it instinctively; for some it is foreign and hard to get into the flow of. Regardless, we all run to a rhythm, to many rhythms. Within each of us is a unique inner rhythm. It's like our tune. Our very own symphony, our rock or blues band (as you wish)! This band has a rhythm, held, supported, nourished, and enlivened by nature's rhythm.

We establish ourselves in our own innate rhythm by following a daily routine, a pattern, with regularity, as doing so gives constancy and allows processes to flow well. A routine builds up a particular integrity that bestows good health for our energy, clarity, wellness, digestion, menstrual cycles, and overall experience of life.

Although each of us remains uniquely individual, with our own inner biological rhythm, we all resonate with cycles and rhythms of nature. That means each of us thrives by living in ways that are conducive to these inner biological rhythms.

Seasons have different qualities. In some geographic locations, the variations in these qualities are more dramatic than in others, such as a Siberian winter, Himalayan spring, or Australian summer. In other parts of the world, the qualities of each season are subtler, but they do have their own identity and the rhythm varies with each molecule changing in its essence.

The difference in quality is because of the elements that compose each location. Humans also vary in physicality, personality, mental qualities, strengths, weaknesses, and other characteristics. That is why some folk thrive in the tropics and struggle while living in cold, dry climates. Others would crawl into a snow cave any day over the hot, humid sun of the tropics or arid, dry desert.

The key to cycles and seasons is to live in a way that is conducive to remaining inwardly in balance with the external environment and not aggravated or ill-effected by it. Some simple illustrations of this are to go to sleep when the sun goes down and to rise at dawn. Eat seasonal, locally grown foods, adjust your pace of life and activities according to the seasons, like being quieter and more inwardly reflecting, eating warming, heavier foods, and sleeping more in winter. Get the rhythm here?

Cycles of the Day

Within each day there are different rhythms. Ayurvedically, these can be divided into zones where one of each of the three dośas is dominant. Each zone is repeated twice throughout a twenty-four-hour cycle. At each zone, there are also crossover junctions that have heightened movement and flux as the dominant forces change.

Just as each part of a twenty-four-hour cycle has differing qualities, so too do we feel and experience differently in each part of the day. We are kidding ourselves if we think we can subtly feel and remain the same in our internal environment throughout the entirety of twenty-four hours. We cannot. We fluctuate, for this is our very nature. Yet when we understand what these fluctuations are, we can still thrive and have great vitality while living through the junctions of each day. We develop awareness as our bodies subtly readjust themselves and recalibrate to meet the dominant rhythm of the changing phases of each zone.

From dawn to when the sun is getting high in the sky, at about 10 a.m., we are in a kapha-dominant phase of day. This means there is more heaviness and dampness in the atmosphere and our digestion is slower, heavier. Mucus and phlegm can be felt more in the body at this time. This is why if you have cough or cold, there will be more mucus production at this time of day. I am sure many of you can relate to waking up with a snotty nose or phlegm in the throat, which shifts and subsides as the day goes on and the pitta forces become stronger. Finding it hard to wake up although having had a long sleep can also be due to kapha elements being dominant at this time of day.

From midmorning to midafternoon, 10 a.m. to 3 p.m., the sun is at its highest and your digestion is at its strongest. This is a pitta-dominant time of day. This is why people who skip breakfast, or even those who have eaten, have an "all gone" feeling in the gut at this time of day. The inner fire may be too stoked, and you may be ravenously hungry for more fuel to keep it burning. The element of warmth is much stronger at this phase of the day. This is the time you can digest the biggest meal, although in Western culture we have it back to front, often skipping our midday meal, not eating enough substance and sustenance, then eating a large meal in the evening.

Midafternoon to early evening, 3 p.m. to 7 p.m., is when vata and movement become dominant. Here we can see energy drop, and a late afternoon "cuppa" and snack are often needed to replenish and boost us. For many it can be an unsettling, even melancholic, time of day.

This is actually the time of day when coffee is most therapeutic. Many people who drink coffee or tea will have it first thing in the morning. It's a great ritual and I love it myself. However, it's not really the optimal time of day to have these stimulating beverages. In the morning, our energy is naturally more refreshed and renewed, so we do not therapeutically require the boost that caffeinated drinks give us. In the afternoon, during the vata junction, energy can wane, and this is a time to give it the appreciated booster.

The kapha, pitta, and vata zones then repeat themselves, and this is our twenty-four-hour cycle. I encourage lifestyle habits that support you and give optimal life energy and wellness by living more in synchronicity with these phases of the day.

Many people find it difficult to get to sleep in the evening, are still awake at 1 a.m., or they wake at 4 a.m. and cannot get back to sleep. It can be as simple as getting into the rhythms and patterns of the day that support you through these sleep patterns, particularly the flux of each junction from zone to zone.

Waking at 4 a.m. and not being able to get to sleep again is indicative that you are being affected by the vata phase of predawn hours. This is when inner movement is heightened, as it is in nature. Keeping this inner movement and your *vāyu*, or inner wind, pacified allows you to be less affected and not to be wakened as this part of the daily cycle comes into being.

From 10 p.m. onward is a time when pitta is dominant. It's strong again as inwardly more energy is produced for the many digestive processes taking place. You may feel more physically or mentally stimulated with a surge of energy if you are not already in bed. Your inner headquarters and key organ of discrimination, the liver, is working hard to enliven the blood at this time. It's working hard for you and needs you to be resting so it can do its vital job efficiently.

You are constantly moving with the daily cycles of nature and your inner rhythms are constantly affected by them. When you work and flow with them, you feel well and clear. Just as when you live against them and you fall out of synchronicity, you feel the consequences.

Just as your physical body has physiological rhythms you can touch, feel, and observe, so, too, does your feeling body, the body of your vitality, and your all-knowing body that resides in the hub of your very being. This is the rhythm of your soul body.

Establish a Daily Rhythm

Here are the keys to establishing a daily routine for you as a woman, and for people of all ages:

1. Wake up at a similar time each day. This establishes an internal pattern in which you can thrive. If you are getting up at a different time each day, the body becomes somewhat confused and constantly has to adjust itself. Cows do not do that. Birds like roosters do not vary in their waking times. Flowers open and bloom when the sun is up and shining, and so do humans. Establishing yourself in a rising pattern season upon season, year upon year bestows equanimity.

2. Spend time outdoors in the morning light (whether the sun is shining or not) for ten to twenty minutes. This is metabolic bliss. Dr. Nancy Lonsdorf, Integrative Medicine physician and Ayurvedic doctor, says research shows that people who do this daily have up to 20 percent less body weight. It is the light that is important for us. Metabolically it is working in a way that is important for our longevity.

3. Eat meals at a similar time each day. Skipping meals or eating meals at constantly varying times makes it hard for digestion to keep up and do the best it possibly can. If you are used to eating lunch at noon, then try to consistently eat between 11:30 a.m. and 1 p.m. every day. Varying this regularly, chopping and changing, makes it really confusing for your gut. If chopping and changing one's mind is challenging for you, imagine the mind of your gut when dealing with this on a regular basis! Support your "gut brain" by eating meals at regular times daily.

4. Go to bed at a similar time each evening. Yes, of course, on the weekend you may stay up later, socializing with family or friends, watching a movie, or celebrating. However, the more you establish a sleeping pattern in which you thrive, the more you will cultivate within you an innate desire to go to bed at a similar time. This may dampen your party style, but hey, brunch or afternoon tea parties are truly good fun and you can still go to

bed early. I love social celebrations in the earlier part of the day, especially when I still get the space at the end of my day to digest the occasion in its entirety, sleep well, and let go the effects of it so that I don't carry it into tomorrow in a way that depletes me. The chapter 9, on sleep, goes into more detail about establishing good sleeping patterns and habits.

You can see where rhythms play out in your life daily by looking at your daily patterns and habits. Just as we can cultivate health-promoting habits that support us rhythmically, we can also develop daily habits that feed imbalance. How do you know which is benefiting you and which may be holding you back?

Well, self-enquiry and reflection will give you the answers. I ask myself the following questions, and I encourage you to ask them of yourself, too:

- How are you feeling within yourself?

- Does your body feel light and energetic, with freedom of movement and without aches or pains?

- Is your body working well for you?

- Are you feeling mentally stable and emotionally balanced? Are you stressed, reactive, emotionally oversensitive, and unable to create or think clearly?

- Is your gut function the best you believe it can be? Truly, is it?

- Are you sleeping well? Is your sleep refreshing?

I believe you need to check in with yourself and be honest in your answers. If nothing else, practice a consistent daily routine and you will experience change within yourself.

My teacher in pulse reading, Dr. Pankaj Naram, would say, "If you keep doing what you are doing, you will keep getting what you are getting." Well, ain't that the truth!

Regularity and routine will hold you in a rhythm in which you can thrive for all your life. This is the substance of the very inner architecture in which your most subtle feeling and mental bodies can thrive. Dear woman, I cannot overestimate the golden forces these keys possess for your wellness.

CHAPTER 6

Hormones and Metabolic Health

. . . .

WOMEN ARE MORE pitta-dominant than men because of the female reproductive hormones. Hormones are complex and intricate. However, in the simplest context, we all have two kinds of hormones: those that relate to reproductive health or sex hormones, and those that relate to base metabolic survival or stress hormones.

These two sets of hormones must remain nourished throughout all the phases and transitions of life. As women, we know this can be especially challenging with the cyclic fluctuations, surges, and changes to female reproductive hormones through the course of life.

Women also have an extra channel in the body, the lactation channel. This channel gives us the ability to produce milk to feed a baby. This channel draws from a woman's rasa dhātu, or her lymph and plasma, hence the importance of keeping your juices hydrated, fed, and flavorsome. These juices are what give your life its flavor.

If you draw too much on your survival hormones throughout your life, then at the time of perimenopause, imbalance starts to show itself. Further, at the cessation of your cycle, when the reproductive hormones diminish, you will be depleted and can have health problems.

If you are hormonally balanced, then when these reproductive hormones lessen, you will still have enough nourishment housed in the survival hormones to stay well, vital, and strong. This means you can navigate the menopausal transition without disharmony and discomfort.

Synthetic hormones further deplete the survival hormones, leading to many different health problems. Hormonal creams are used to balance hormones that change too rapidly and with extremes. Hormonal creams are effective and do give relief but, again, what's really needed is to pacify what is behind the extreme hormonal shifts.

First, any treatment that will be effective, deep, and permanent has to address and pacify vata in all aspects of your physiology and being. Unless a hormonal cream or treatment energetically addresses and pacifies vata, and typically synthetic hormonal treatments do not, then they are merely a bandage. A few natural hormonal creams address the management of vata; however, a cream alone is not a long-term panacea to disturbances.

It's tough and overwhelming to experience a hormonal imbalance. It compounds the stress you're already experiencing in your entire being. When sleep is disturbed because of aggravated metabolic processes, and the condition becomes chronic, then life can become weary, heavy, and overwhelming. There can be depression, anxiety, emotional sensitivity, and overactivity. The mental channels become strained and aggravated. The body experiences weariness and intense fatigue. Yet the demands of life placed upon a woman remain the same and do not compensate her for the hormonal shifts that are creating absolute internal chaos in her life.

Hormone Replacement Therapy
....

Hormone replacement therapy is not a healing solution to a woman's health challenge. It will manage symptoms but cannot address the underlying imbalance. It is synthetic and warming, and it affects the overall metabolic function of the entire being.

Although complaints can be so troublesome for women, impacting significantly the quality of life, hormonal substitution is a shortsighted solution. Yes, it relieves women of symptoms of discomfort from hormonal imbalance in the short term. However, it keeps the life forces of a woman bound up in the reproductive processes and, therefore, unable to be released for spiritual activity, as is the natural shift at this time of change in a woman's hormones.

HORMONES IMBALANCES

Patients commonly ask me if their hormones are imbalanced. It has been my clinical experience that women generally know when their hormones are imbalanced. What they do not know is *how* to balance them.

Not knowing the *how* and *what* is disempowering. Remember, you were created by the divine to experience empowerment, so let's learn how to balance your metabolic function. You start by addressing the equilibrium in your life, bolstering your digestion and then your rhythms as the basis for healthy metabolic processes.

You need to look at your whole lifestyle and balance your hormones if you are feeling dull, flat, heavy, foggy, uncertain, confused, unmotivated; if you're not sleeping well, have menstrual difficulty or changing patterns and fluctuations of your menstrual cycle; if you are irritable, overemotional, generally feeling like crap and like life feels hard constantly; or if you are making life hard for those close to you.

Know that you can always do something about this. Although you cannot do everything at once, you can always take gentle, small, specific steps and do *something*.

For example, look at your diet in the context of cycles and rhythms. Are you eating at regular meal times daily? What kinds of food are you eating? What time are you going to bed? Are you making time for inner reflection and nourishment daily? I encourage you to consider all these elements, to reflect upon them periodically. It's like doing an inventory of the most precious house you will ever dwell in.

CHAPTER 7

Exercise

. . . .

BECAUSE OUR BODIES have so many gross and subtle moving parts, it is pretty obvious that we are designed to move. In order to keep the moving parts limber, we need to move regularly.

Movement creates metabolic bliss, which means optimal functioning of all chemical processes of each organism. However, we fare well to be educated as women about the kinds of exercise that are beneficial to our longevity. Constitutionally, each body type benefits most from the kind of exercise that complements and supports its inherent nature.

If you think about the qualities of the dośas, then you can start to get an understanding and image of the kinds of exercise that can benefit or aggravate a person.

Vata, being energy that is light, erratic, and spent all at once in bursts with no reserve or moderation, is nourished by gentle exercise. Walking, hatha yoga, tai chi, gentle paddling, and yin yoga are among the kinds of exercise that support a person with this kind of constitution. Overexercising and overstimulation will ultimately deplete and further imbalance a vata-dominant woman. And, if you are called to do strong exercise and you are a vata type, then be clever. Support and nourish yourself with lifestyle, diet, and all the tools and home remedies to keep you as well as can be in your activities.

> Susie, age forty-seven, was experiencing joint pain, hip and back stiffness, bloating and erratic appetite, constipation, poor sleep, and anxiety. Her work as a yoga teacher meant her schedule was erratic and it was difficult to establish regular mealtimes. She felt her body ought to be stronger, have more capacity to "keep up" with her schedule, and experience better digestion and flexibility. She was, however, vata-aggravated. Her body was internally dry. She was perimenopausal and her hormonal secretions were drying up too quickly. She needed unctuous pacifying, lubricating, and gentle nourishment.
>
> I gave her a diet that was easily digestible so that she could bolster her digestion and take suitable foods and meals in a rhythmical, regular way around her teaching schedule. I also gave her herbal remedies. I recommended a daily self-oil massage with warmed sesame oil. I suggested she incorporate more restorative yoga āsana in her own practice. This was key for her, to do gentle, slow, rejuvenating exercise that created the space to pacify her nervous system, circulatory system, digestive system, organs, and mental channels. The restorative, gentle exercise was necessary to realign her inner equilibrium.
>
> Although it was initially challenging for her to establish a regular daily routine incorporating the recommendations, she did, and they quickly became easy for her because she was more internally nourished and lubricated. The joint pain and stiffness disappeared, and she felt strength and freedom in her body. Her digestion improved, regulating her appetite and healthy bowel movements. Her sleep improved and she no longer experienced anxiety. The condition of her entire being improved dramatically with these simple practices.

Pitta has more capacity, grit, and endurance, and people with a pitta constitution can do more intense exercise. The thing to be mindful of with pitta is that it is driven and motivated, sharp and penetrating. Pitta seeks the challenge and has the capability; however, it can be overstimulated and there can be a hunger for ever-greater challenges. There is a time to pull back and be moderate, otherwise one can become too intensely driven to accomplish. Heat will aggravate, so it is not recommended to run a marathon in the high noon sun nor do headstands and hot yoga in the late morning to early afternoon.

> Rose, age forty-two, is a mental health nurse. She came to see me for reflux, loose stools, skin rashes, excessive sweating of her hands and feet, and hair loss. Rose surfed, cycled, and did yoga āsana daily. Sometimes she cycled thirty-plus miles, surfed, and did a "vigorous" yoga practice, all before mid-morning. And, if not working a shift that day, she would do it all again in the afternoon. The more exercise the better. Even when physically fatigued, with aches and pains (which were coming up more regularly), she was driven to exercise hard. She would feel irritation and intense emotions if anyone or anything got in the way of her daily exercise.
>
> Rose was high pitta and had excessive metabolic heat. It was creating inflammation in her gut and digestive organs, channels of elimination, and mental channels.
>
> In addition to a diet to pacify pitta (avoiding sour and fermented foods) and herbal remedies, we looked at Rose's lifestyle. We worked to bring a more moderate approach to her exercise. Although she was keen to continue with all her activities, she avoided doing stimulating exercise in the heat of the day, from 11 a.m. to 2 p.m., particularly in the warmer seasons.
>
> In pacifying Rose's excess pitta, she was able to develop more discrimination and could be softer, less intense, and more discerning about her exercise regime. She became more moderate. Her passion was greater than ever but what shifted was her ability to perceive what really supported her body and being, for greater immediate vitality and longevity. Of course, her digestion improved too!

Kapha by nature is slow and steady. It is also heavy. People with more kapha tend to have heavier bodies, slower metabolism, and sometimes an aversion to moving their bodies. This can be perceived as laziness. It can certainly create sluggishness. So kapha needs to be stimulated. Although slow to get going, once on the move, these people have good staying power.

Jean, age forty-six, is a biodynamic farmer. She came to see me because, although she moved her body regularly during her physical labor as a farmer, ate wholesome, nutritious, seasonal food, and not too much of it, she was overweight. It did not matter what kind of diet she tried, she'd been unsuccessful in shedding the excess pounds. Each time she worked hard to lose a few pounds, she'd yo-yo and gain even more. She also served on a local governance board and had endured considerable stress in recent years in this position of service.

Jean had an abundance of kapha by her very nature. This made her a wonderfully nourishing, steady person who, although slow to get started, was most persistent and had the staying power to ensure the job was done. She also had good pitta. This meant that she naturally tends to accumulate and retain, as she had slow metabolism.

I recommended she move her body in the morning to stimulate her metabolism. She began a routine of starting her morning with meditation practices and reflection space followed by fifteen to twenty minutes of brisk walking.

She drank ginger tea in the morning to stimulate her digestion before eating a light breakfast with stimulating spices, including cinnamon and ginger. She did not take her next meal until four to five hours later. Likewise with her evening meal. To remove the retention of excess fluid in her body, Jean avoided tomatoes and yogurt, and kept grains to only 15 to 20 percent of her daily intake. Therefore, if she ate grain for lunch, she did not eat them at breakfast or dinner. This way of eating supported her slow metabolism to recalibrate itself optimally. She also would regularly start the day with vegetable or mung soup for breakfast and not eat again until her noon meal. Once a week, she did a mung soup cleanse day not only to remove the excess of fluid she was retaining but to bolster digestion and support the elimination of accumulation in the tissues.

Not only did following the above recommendations boost Jean's slow metabolism, but she slowly and steadily lost the excess pounds she'd been carrying, giving her more physical energy, better quality of sleep, and greater productivity. She was able to understand her nature more fully, recognizing that she cringed and retreated into herself when confronted with stress and conflict, which she had been doing in her position on the local governance board. By stimulating her digestion and metabolism, pacifying both her pitta and excess kapha doṡas, in her position Jean was able to find her voice and articulate clearly her feelings and concepts. She was able to respond and rise to the occasion with integrity in herself.

CHAPTER 8

Food

. . . .

WHERE DO I begin to write about food? Perhaps with a blessing on our food. A blessing and gratitude to Mother Earth, who grew the food in all her elements. To the farmers, those who harvest, pack, and transport food to the points of purchase. To the abundance and variety of food available to us. Living in Australia, my family and I are so privileged to have good quality air, water, and access to fresh, clean, whole foods. We have good resources available to learn about food.

However, there can be so much information available about food, much of it varied and conflicting, that it becomes stressful and confusing to know what food to eat. When this happens, people are eating the food of stress and confusion. Believe me, this is indigestible. Tuning in to the nature of food, aligning to your nature, makes it possible to understand and eat the food of love and vitality.

Ayurveda looks at food from an energetic perspective. That means the energetic qualities of a food are considered in how they influence the dośas.

Appendix B contains recommendations about how to eat, including eating in a conducive environment in which you focus fully on your food without multitasking. Cultivate a ritual and a blessing around your meal, as mentioned in chapter 3, on digestion.

As much as possible, keep your food fresh, local, and grown as close to nature as possible. Avoid processed foods, refined sugars, and leftover foods as much as possible. Understand that your food is a sacred gift to give you strength so that you can be of contribution and know yourself.

Eating and Food in Contemporary Life

My children's community school, since its inception, has held a monthly "chai café" for children, families, teachers, and friends to gather and share our blessings over chai and food. I recall fondly that, in the early years, one mother brought a huge watermelon and the children devoured it. Like a magic pudding, there was enough for all. All the children could share in the eating of this offering. Over the years, as the community grew, allergies and aversions grew, sensitivities and unmet needs grew; so, too, did the format and offering of the foods served. An array of gluten-free foods appeared, and listing ingredients became necessary. Sugar-free, dairy-free, nut-free. Fortunately, never love-free! For me, something so pure, generous, and full in spirit became a complicated business. One day, my youngest daughter, who was three at the time, looked up innocently while in the serving line of the community café and asked, "Mum, am I allowed to eat gluten?" I could not believe my three-year-old child even possessed such a word in her vocabulary.

My questions to you are, "Why are you eating a particular food?" and "Why are you not eating a particular food?" They're open questions, posed for open contemplation.

Con pane. "With bread," a companion. Bread is made in the essence and spirit of offering, sharing, and eating together with love. When received in the right context, with the right understanding, this substance becomes healing nourishment to the human being's organism. Now, hang on to your hat, dear woman. I have not mentioned the grain in the bread. I've simply said "bread"!

Dr. Rudolf Steiner, who introduced the living life processes, in a lecture in Dornach, Switzerland, in 1920, said this of diet, because he knew that it was a question of the social aspect of the human being, not only the medical: "We could spend a long time debating the significance and validity of various peculiar diets, but the main consideration is that any dietary restriction makes people antisocial. This is where the social and medical aspects collide."

It is my observation and clinical experience that people have a wish to find their place in the world, to experience and fulfill a fundamental human need for connection. To belong in a community, in a tribe, in a circle of like-minded people, in a family. Hence the constant seeking and striving to fit in. Children, in particular, wish to be a part of the whole and belong. It is an innate yearning.

Dr. Steiner says the significance of the Last Supper was not that Christ gave each disciple something special, but that he gave them all the same thing. The possibility of coming together with others to eat or drink is of great social significance, and anything that tends to interfere with this healthy social aspect of our human nature needs to be handled with some caution.

Take care that you're not developing likes and aversions, not only on a conscious level of being but on an organic level internally as well. The digestive process physically, mentally, and emotionally can be influenced by such likes and dislikes.

Your thoughts have a far more immediate biological effect on your physiology than the food you eat. Thoughts affect the tissues much faster than the metabolic processes of food ingested. Truly food for thought.

We can lose the inherent capacity to overcome. Resilience is weakened. Eating, and understanding our digestive processes, calls for discernment.

Remember: everything in moderation. Not too little, nor too much. Balance. Partake in life, in social engagement in a wholesome, balanced way for good health of the entire being.

CHAPTER 9

Sleep

· · · · · · · · · · · · ·

THE MORE I learn as a woman, health practitioner, and mother, the more I appreciate the fundamental wisdom imparted in simply teaching our children to eat and sleep well. These are the basic building blocks for wellness.

Why is it so important to teach our children to sleep well? Sleep is a foundation for good health for them, which is imparted through life and imprinted as adults. Children follow and imitate rhythms, so if adults know how to sleep well, then children follow suit. Bedtime is bedtime! Give it as much importance as other activities of your day.

It is a blessing to look forward to going to sleep each night so that I can rise and begin a new day. Looking forward to bedtime for some, however, is not a given. So many obstacles prohibit a lot of people from going to bed at a reasonable hour and from getting adequate rest. These could be working hours; family commitments; having to watch that movie that was recommended, listening to that podcast, attending that webinar, reading the paper, which there was no time for in the day, checking one more social media message, searching and becoming engrossed on the internet; working too late; catching up on household chores; even having some quiet time to contemplate the busyness of your day. The list is endless and individual. However, often obstacles are simply habits that keep you from going to bed.

For some people, the thought of going to sleep is traumatic. For some, sleep just does not come easily. Negative, worrying thoughts dance and swirl, creating unrest, unease, and uncomfortable dreams. There is a plethora of scenarios that stop people from embracing bedtime, which could come so naturally at the end of a day. For a person with chronic insomnia, going to bed is arduous and exhausting, not necessarily something to be savored.

Vital functions take place in sleep. While we slumber, many processes involving complex metabolic actions occur. Having gone through the day engaged in intricate processes of breaking down and metabolizing, our liver now builds up metabolic processes, strength, and capacity to be a joyful, discerning being again. Hence a certain amount of stimulating energy is released in the body. This energy is not designed to be spent in other processes but is used primarily for maintaining and sustaining our wellness in all aspects of our being. When this process occurs without interference, physical, mental, emotional, and spiritual discrimination and discretion are imparted with clarity of being.

When we sleep, our subtle "feeling body" actually travels to a place where we receive spiritual nourishment, an essence required to carry out our worldly tasks the following day. We require deep sleep to receive this subtle nourishment.

Vata needs deep sleep in order to be pacified. Pitta needs good rest and sleep in order to be pacified. Kapha has the tendency and nature to sleep a lot, as we do in early childhood years. In adulthood, however, a person with kapha dominance has to be mindful not to oversleep. Digestion needs good rest for metabolic processes to be robust and flowing.

Sleep is a pillar for wellness in all aspects of how we live. In my clinic and while teaching, I tell people that what they simply need is routine and rhythm. I usually share simple foundational rules and at the top of the list is sleep. The quality of your sleep equates to the quality of your life. It affects your relationships, work, energy, and enthusiasm.

While you are awake, you receive nourishment from many sources: the sun, the food you eat, your daily tasks, and your relationships. While you are asleep, you receive spiritual nourishment from a cosmic source. This kind of subtle nourishment fuels you to fulfill your life's work the following day on awakening. It is a particular type of fuel that can only be received and taken up if you sleep deeply and long enough to receive it.

When you do not get good sleep, you can experience immediate effects: weariness, fatigue, lack of clarity and focus; dullness, heaviness, grumpiness and downright irritability; short, sharp, emotional and erratic reactions, instead of modulated responses.

We can make poor choices to immediately alleviate the feeling from lack of sleep, such as eating foods that give instant energy but follow with heaviness and emptiness or consuming caffeine-loaded drinks. However, all that's needed is simply rest.

Sleeping Patterns

Depending on our innate bodily constitutions or types, we have different sleep patterns. We repeatedly come in and out of sleep cycles during the course of a night's sleep. A sleep cycle means that you naturally come into a lighter sleep and then go deep again; it does not mean you will wake. For vata-dominant people, the cycle is 1.5 hours. For pitta-dominant folk, it's 2.5 hours, and kapha-dominant people have a 3-hour cycle. However, if disturbed for any reason or weak in digestive capacity, then you might awaken, or you may naturally wake up and rise at different times than other people. It is natural for you and you will serve yourself well to honor this rhythm. To wake naturally is the best tonic, as opposed to being woken up by an alarm. If you need to wake at 7 a.m. and naturally wake at 6:20 a.m., before the alarm goes off, then you have come out of a sleep cycle. Get up. If you go back to sleep and wake up forty minutes later artificially, then you wake mid-sleep cycle and will not have the natural energy reserves you otherwise would have by getting up earlier, but naturally.

Naps and sleeps during the day are best avoided unless you are ill, convalescing, preparing for shift work or napping with an infant or young child (a must). The reason naps are generally discouraged is because day sleep interferes with digestive processes. Heaviness and mucus-like sludge can accumulate in the body when we day nap. If you do feel called to rest during the day, particularly after having eaten a meal, then lie on your left side to support your digestive processes.

Sleeping Positions

When going to sleep, it is best initially to lie on your left side for fifteen to twenty minutes. This position encourages the best internal movement and digestive flow in the body. Then you can lie on your back or in a preferred sleeping position.

Tips to Encourage Good Sleep

To encourage a good night's rest, try incorporating some or all of the following techniques:

1. Massage ghee into your temples before bed. This substance is pacifying and calming to the small but important nerves and vessels that become overstimulated and stretched by your day.

2. When you have not slept well or enough, it is also nourishing and therapeutic to massage ghee around the eyes to pacify the local nerves and vessels.

3. Massage ghee or warmed sesame oil into the soles of your feet before bed.

4. A hot milk spiced with cinnamon, cardamom, fennel, and a little turmeric powder is a nourishing tonic to promote good sleep. If you are able to tolerate cow's milk, then organic, unhomogenized is recommended. Whatever your choice, be it dairy, soy, oat, almond, or rice milk, make it hot and make it spiced!

5. According to the principles of Vastu (the ancient Hindu science of energy principles of the universe applied to the architecture of the body), the head should be facing south or east for good sleep. Why not to the north? The energetic effect of the North Pole draws the iron forces of the body to the head, which can create unrefreshing, unsettling, disturbing dreams and sleep.

   The bedroom should be uncluttered, ideally without electronic devices like TVs or computers. It is best not to have mirrors facing the bed. Essentially the bedroom is a room of quietude.

6. Get up at the same time each morning.

7. Go outside in the morning for the light, every day, even if it's winter or cloudy. This light supports metabolism.

8. Refrain from any kind of screen time, including your phone, for thirty minutes before sleep.

9. If you use your phone as an alarm, switch it to airplane mode when you go to bed. If you do not need your phone as an alarm, then do not keep it in the bedroom while you sleep.

10. Draw your curtains and do what you can to ensure your room is as quiet and dark as possible. Use an eye mask if your room is affected by light from street lamps and the like.

11. Take a foot bath or bath with lavender oil and/or Epsom salts.

12. Consider supportive and effective Ayurvedic herbal remedies to support your quality of sleep. I recommend Ayushakti
Sumedha or Ayushakti Blis formula, as prescribed by an Ayurvedic practitioner, or the anthroposophical homeopathic remedy
Bryophyllum.

You cannot put fuel in the car if you do not stop at the pump
and remain stationary long enough to fill the tank. Just as if you
put the wrong fuel in the car, it would not run to its best capacity.
It may cough, splutter, and even break down.

Sleep and the Dośa

**Sleep is the most effective way to manage stress hormones.
Sleep is necessary for your ongoing good metabolic function.
Sleep is necessary for nourishment on all levels of your being.**

How much sleep is enough? How do you know if sleep is deep
enough?

In the different phases of life, varying amounts of sleep are
needed to nourish, sustain, and thrive. Within this, there are slight
variations for different constitutions. A child who is more vata dominant will generally sleep less than a child who is kapha dominant.
The vata-dominant child will waken early in the morning, often
predawn, full of beans and mental energy, and ready to go. The
kapha-dominant child will feel heavy, sluggish, and slow to start. This
characteristic is relevant not only in childhood but throughout life.
The fact is, we have night owls and we have larks!

In the kapha-dominant phase of life, from childhood to sixteen to
eighteen years old, inherently more sleep is needed to build the body
with all the earth forces required to make the physical architecture
strong so that we can embody the spiritual forces of our beings. Kids
just need more sleep.

In the pitta-dominant phase of life, typically from ages sixteen to fifty, we still need good sleep and seven to eight hours of sleep is the basic golden amount required for wellness. The above principles still apply, up until fifty-plus years of age. In this phase of life, we have more life forces to create, drive, and manifest, and we are able to survive and function with less sleep. Obviously, nature created things this way or parents of young children would simply buckle from sheer lack of good sleep!

When people have difficulty sleeping or insomnia, there are usually contributing factors. Insomnia is the inability to sleep or habitual sleeplessness. It is my understanding that true insomnia occurs in a small percentage of people. The underlying root cause for the majority of people experiencing sleep difficulties is anxiety. Excessive worry increases when going to bed, making deep sleep even harder to gain. Other causes include physical pain, joint pain, urinary and prostate conditions. When we address and deal with these conditions, the quality of sleep can improve.

However, for people to experience good-quality sleep, they need to pacify the force of vata. When vāyu is going up to the head and creating excessive activity in the nerve sensory and mental channels, it needs to be pacified and brought back down into the organs of metabolism, for better sleep.

This pacifying effect not only allows a gentleness in the mental channels that is needed for sleep to occur, but it also supports good digestion, which equates to a better quality of sleep. When quality sleep supports digestive processes, hormonal function is more aligned and stronger, which means better sleep. Excess metabolic heat can then be pacified through the cooling nourishment and activity of sleep. Finally, accumulation in all the channels of the mind, the emotional body, and all tissues and organs can be reduced, which improves the quality of sleep. Simply remember the establishment of good sleep patterns for a child—these are to be reestablished in you for a healthy adulthood.

Particularly as you age, all of the above is of utmost significance. In the third phase of your life, when vata doṣa, internal wind and air, becomes dominant by nature, sleep patterns will be more sensitive and irregular unless harmonized and pacified—anchored within you.

I encourage you to seek ways of actively supporting your quality of sleep so that you can be fully alive in your waking hours, dear woman. You've got important tasks to fulfill!

CHAPTER 10

Breathing

· · · · · · · · · · · ·

OUR LIFE BEGINS and ends with breath. The average woman breathes about 21,600 times a day.

Conceptually, I've always understood the importance of good breathing. Consciously, I've not been so consistent in practicing it with disciplined focus and awareness. Several years ago, I was in a workshop and the facilitator asked me how much time I spend focusing on my breathing every day. He said that if it was only during meditation practice, then I was selling myself short. What about the rest of the day?

Dr. Rudolf Steiner reiterated the significance of a parent's role in teaching children to eat, sleep, and breathe well, which always resonates deeply. *Of course*, it is beneficial to one's entire being to breathe well.

Clinically, I've always marveled at patients who have had exceptional breakthroughs and improvements with health challenges of all kinds by working with their breathing techniques.

Prāṇāyāma

Prāṇāyāma lifts the veil of ignorance from the Inner Light.
THE YOGA SUTRAS OF PATANJALI, 2.52

"Prāṇa" is the Sanskrit word for breath, the vital life force. *Yāma* means to control or restrain.

Prāṇāyāma practice is the controlled practice of breathing. According to Vedic texts, the ancient yogis understood that when we control our breath, we control our state of mind. If we change our breathing patterns, our mental and emotional state can change. Such states are the root of all physical ailments, and so people's health challenges shift and improve when they work with purposefully controlling their breathing patterns.

I've had an interesting relationship to prāṇāyāma practice over the years. In yoga classes, I would yearn for it and yet wrestle with mental resistance and very mediocre mind chatter when actually doing it. Why?

It was only recently that I had a physical experience and a realization that for most of my adult life, I've breathed against the flow of the universe instead of allowing the universe and life to "breathe" me. Phew! Thankfully there's still time to work that one out.

Prāṇāyāma has varying effects on our body and mind because it works on and purifies the nervous system. It can support the body to strengthen the "switch" from the sympathetic (active) to the parasympathetic (rest and digest) nervous system. Prāṇāyāma supports the body to more readily and easily be in a rested, relaxed state of being.

Prāṇāyāma is the fourth of the eight limbs of yoga. It is defined by T.K.V. Desikachar in his classic text *The Heart of Yoga* as "the conscious, deliberate regulation of the breath replacing unconscious patterns of breathing."

Because prāṇāyāma is effective and works on the nervous system and with it you are consciously controlling subtle rhythms of breathing, I recommend working with a qualified, experienced practitioner of yoga and prāṇāyāma to learn the many different kinds of breathing techniques.

Two Types of Breath

Two common prāṇāyāma practices that you may be familiar with are *ujjayi* breath and alternate nostril breathing.

UJJAYI BREATHING
Here are the steps for ujjayi breath:

1. As you exhale, slightly constrict the bottom of your throat, making a *haaaa* sound, as if fogging up glass with the moisture from your breath.

2. As you inhale, make the same sound.

3. Breathe through your nose with your mouth closed with this sound.

4. Extend your inhale by slowly counting to five.

5. As you exhale slowly count to five.

6. Make your inhale and exhale smooth and of equal length and intensity.

7. Inhale and then exhale five times in this way.

ALTERNATE NOSTRIL BREATHING
The steps for alternate nostril breathing are as follows:

1. Hold up your right-hand palm facing you with your first two fingers bent and your thumb, ring finger, and little finger straight.

2. Close your mouth.

3. Lightly press your ring finger on the left side of your nose, closing your left nostril.

4. Inhale through your right nostril for a slow count of five.

5. Release your ring finger from your left nostril.

6. Lightly press your thumb on the right side of your nose, closing your right nostril.

7. Exhale through your left nostril for a slow count of five.

8. With your thumb still holding the right nostril shut, inhale through the left nostril for a slow count of five.

9. Release your thumb from your right nostril.

10. Again, press your ring finger on the left side of your nose, closing your left nostril. Exhale through your right nostril for a slow count of five.

11. One round is composed of an inhale right, exhale left, inhale left, exhale right.

12. Repeat for three rounds.

CHAPTER 11

Cleansing

· · · · · · · · · · · ·

SINCE TIME IMMEMORIAL, ancients cleansed to get closer to their innate source of self and to realize their true nature. We cleanse to relieve ourselves of the burdens acquired through living—the challenges and accumulations of being in a human body. We cleanse to recalibrate and rejuvenate. We cleanse to bring renewal to our life energy. In essence, cleansing fine-tunes us so that we can hear the sound of our own inner music.

Let's look more fully at why cleansing is important for aspects of our being.

Cleansing balances and reconnects us to our heart of truth. It removes fatigue, relieves worry and fear, and gives clarity, purpose, and ease.

Cleansing creates lightness in our body and being. It removes excess gas, water, heaviness, bulkiness, and sludge. It removes retention, swelling, and dullness. It not only creates a physical spaciousness, but it also promotes a better-quality sleep, greater mental clarity, courage, and focus. We are able to respond better to life rather than perpetually living in a state of knee-jerk reactiveness. When we cleanse, we relieve the load on all aspects of our being.

Ayurveda has one of the most ancient yet sophisticated, simple, and effective ways to cleanse the tissues, channels, organs, emotions, patterns, and ruts that impede your soul's passage.

What is the sound of your tissues? What is the sound of your channels? Can you hear them? Do you listen to them? What are they telling you? Your tissues all have a sound, your heart space has a sound—the sound of your womanhood.

Sufi musician and mystic Hazrat Inayat Khan says that every nerve has its own vibration, which we may call its sound.

Beautiful woman, how do you recognize this sound? How do you hear this sound in the depths of your being? To hear this sound, you cleanse. You clear the path.

We cleanse so that our body may be healed, our mind fortified, and our soul illumined by the grace of God—whether the universe, Mother Earth, spirit, or the divine. We cleanse so that our heart may be made our divine temple. We cleanse to stay well and happy in life and in the light of God, the divine creative force. We cleanse to be a vessel that can hold and flourish in all our wisdom so that we may best fulfill our life's purpose. We cleanse to experience our radiance.

When we cleanse, we rekindle our digestive capacity and function. We optimize our metabolic function and hormonal processes. Cleansing removes fatigue, giving clarity, purpose, ease, and renewal.

Before going deeper into the practicalities of cleansing I suggest you do Enrichment Activity #6 in appendix F, a reflective listening exercise.

Aam (Ama): Metabolic Sludge

In every Indian home, people meticulously sweep the entrance and pathway daily. We, too, must sweep the pathway of the accumulation of living.

Aam is a metabolic sludge that accumulates in the tissues over time. There is mental aam and there is physical aam. The body has no mechanism to naturally eliminate this substance. In the body's innate compassion, it digests and eliminates as much of this substance as it can. However, over time it accumulates, becoming a burden because it blocks and impedes movement, processes, communication, and flow. It impacts our wellness. We have to clear our paths of this blockage.

When the digestive fire, agni, is weakened, you get indigestion. When you do not fully digest something that you ingest, it leaves a partially digested substance. The body does not know what to do with this partially metabolized substance, and it accumulates in the large intestine, where it putrefies, decays, stinks, and is sticky and heavy. It becomes a toxic sludge like mucus. Aam serves no purpose and has no benefit to the body. It is not required to function well. It moves through circulation with the blood and blocks channels in the body.

When aam blocks channels of elimination, it can create constipation or diarrhea. When it blocks channels of circulation it can lead to arteriosclerosis, thrombosis, or even a heart attack. When it blocks respiratory channels it can create sinusitis, asthma, or bronchial complaints. When aam blocks the mental channels it creates confusion, fear, lack of focus, poor concentration, excessive worry, and irritability. Emotionally it can create oversensitivity, feelings of lack, and depression.

Aam can affect your physical vitality and enthusiasm for life. It can affect the quality of your soul life.

Your digestion is how you experience and perceive your life. Your mental channels are so fine and subtle that if they are clogged or resonating too high or low, too hot or cool, too rough or soft, they can become disharmonious and solidly disheartening. You might try many different techniques to change the quality of your mind-set, but your life may change the way you wish because your digestion needs work and your channels may be clogged and sluggish. The quality of these tissues cannot increase when there is accumulation to be penetrated, mobilized, eliminated, or transmuted.

When your thoughts, feelings, or habits loop repeatedly, with the same thoughts creating the same feelings, actions, and results, then the channels need a good cleanup. Too much aam in your channels, particularly the mental channels, makes it difficult to change the quality of your thoughts; it is similar when you have too much vāyu (air) or pitta (heat). Let me tell you, aam is one sticky, stubborn substance, and you will most definitely keep getting the same qualitative results unless you convert or clean it out.

Cleansing is about cleaning channels to allow processes to operate more efficiently in all aspects of your body and being. Then you can cultivate all that you may be seeking and striving for in your precious life.

Ayurveda is holistic and, to me, this means the entire composition of a person, including the soul and what makes a person unique. Ayurveda considers that your symptoms, physical presentations, and illness are simply showing the state of your inner spiritual condition. Disease is evidence of a lack of equilibrium in parts of your inner life. The source arises from the mental channels of the mind. Cleansing purifies these channels and improves the quality of digestion.

How do you know when your digestion is compromised? One way is to look at your sleep. What is the quality of your sleep? If you are waking up feeling anything less than rested, then some level of your digestive capacity needs attention. This is also true if you are waking up during the night. (But not when you're being woken by a child, or a cat needing to be let out!) Is your tongue coated? Does your family wish to leave the room if you pass wind or use the toilet? Are you burping a lot?

If you are experiencing any of these symptoms, then you can truly benefit by taking an honest look at your digestion.

In Australia, we eat a lot of salad. Perhaps not as much as people do in North America, but on both sides of the world, people typically consume a lot of salad when they want to eat healthier and lighter or to lose weight.

I suggest eating some salad greens on the side of your meal. Preferably oiled and lightly dressed. However, eating a huge plate or bowl of salad as your main meal is hard work for your gut. It is, in fact, a heavy meal to digest, and it takes tremendous digestive power to convert salad into a nourishing substance. This may seem bizarre and I am sure many of you will meet this statement with resistance, but let me assure you that a salad of raw vegetables is heavy to digest. It is full of air and gas, and has a heavy, cold quality.

If you experience bloating of any kind, stiffness in the body, discomfort after eating, gut ailments, whether bloating, cramping, or discomfort, then I invite you to stop eating raw food. You will soon enough see how your gut feels.

Cooked food can be warming, as it possesses a warmth familiar to the rhythm of the digestive ability to transform it. This is somewhat different than a heating food, for example a tomato. Tomatoes are sour, which makes them heating. Ghee and pumpkin are examples of heat-pacifying, or cooling, foods.

All foods have an energy: cooling, heating, dry, unctuous, light, heavy. I am not referring to the six different tastes of foods here. That is something separate again (bitter, astringent, pungent, sweet, sour, salty). What I am referring to here is quality on the organism.

The foods our body benefits from most change with the seasons. In autumn, for example, your body requires more warming foods because in nature it is cooler. Your rhythms will be striving to create a dynamic of health by warming up to adapt to the changing conditions.

Toxins, including environmental toxins, will accumulate when you have not fully digested what you have eaten. You will accumulate this sludge-like substance if you do not fully digest any impression you take in or experience you have.

Your digestion is very compassionate, but it has no natural mechanism to remove accumulated sludge from the organs, tissues, and cells of the body. That is why it is great to regularly do things that improve your digestion, such as drinking ginger tea after meals to support digestion. Ginger tea prevents this metabolic sludge from building up so that you can have dynamic life energy.

The simplest way of preventing this sludge from accumulating in the body is to cleanse periodically. Different cultures have done this since the beginning of time. They have fasting days and periods to bring them closer to the divine, to experience and know their true nature.

Identifying Symptoms of Aam

If you experience any of the following, you may have aam:

- You are regularly confused and lack focus.
- Your stool sinks in the toilet like a stone instead of floating.
- Your stool is stinky and sticky and contains undigested food.
- After eating a meal, you feel heavy, dull, and sleepy.
- You need a tea or coffee to get into your day's work.
- Your body looks swollen, bulky, and heavy or obese.
- You cannot gain weight regardless of how much nutritious food you eat.
- Your tongue is coated with a white film.
- Your skin feels sticky.
- You have low energy regardless of how good your nutrition and how many supplements you take.

Accumulating Aam

There are several ways that you accumulate aam:

- You eat fried or processed food, heavy meat, refined wheat flour, excess sweets and refined sugar, excess raw food, and heavy cheeses.
- You eat regularly without real hunger or appetite.
- You drink too much water and cold drinks with meals.
- You have excessive late nights.

- You have a sedentary lifestyle.
- You are too stressed.
- You regularly consume cold, carbonated, or sugar-rich drinks or ice cream.
- You drink alcohol and take recreational drugs.
- You chronically expose yourself to a stressful lifestyle, pollution, and unhealthy life habits.

Eliminating Aam

There are three primary ways to eliminate aam:

- You bolster your digestion optimally so that a transforming energy that can convert the aam is activated.
- You use penetrating herbal remedies that break up the blocks created by and digest the aam.
- You eliminate aam from the tissue, system, and body through fasting and cleansing methods.

Reducing Aam with Diet

To reduce aam with diet, eat only what you can digest. You can only convert into a nourishing substance what you can digest. Regardless of how nourishing or nutrient-dense a food may be, unless you can digest it well, your body will not fully assimilate it. What the body cannot fully use becomes aam.

Generally, a higher ratio of vegetables, especially leafy greens, can be taken in the daily diet, compared with protein and carbs. Keep vegetables (and fruits) daily intake to at least 40 percent.

FOODS TO AVOID

Avoid meat, wheat, refined sugars and excessive sweets, fried food, fermented food, heavy beans (kidney and lima beans, chickpeas), and processed foods.

FOODS TO EAT MORE OFTEN

Eat cooked vegetables, basmati rice, mung soup, split yellow mung dal, and vegetable and fruit juices.

General Eating Habits for Reducing Aam

To reduce aam, cultivate the eating habits that follow:

1. Ayurveda strongly recommends not drinking iced water or refrigerated water during or after a meal. It weakens your agni, or digestive fire. Instead, sip room temperature or warm water.

2. Drinking buttermilk at the end of a meal can support digestion. Buttermilk can be prepared by blending four teaspoons of yogurt with two pinches each of ginger and cumin powder in one cup of water. This buttermilk can be lightly salted or sweetened.

3. Leaving space in the stomach with each meal not only creates room for the dośas and movement of digestive enzymes, it also fosters good digestion and promotes mental clarity. How do you know if you've left space? You may still feel hungry for more, as opposed to full to the gills!

4. Generally, favor eating cooked, warm, soupy meals over cold, dry, solid foods. The warmth of the food stimulates digestive enzymes.

5. Fruits and sweet foods are best eaten separately or before meals. Yes, that does mean dessert before the main. When eaten together, the two are inclined to ferment and disturb digestion of the meal.

6. How much water daily? Ayurveda recommends eight to ten glasses a day in different forms, such as pure water, soups, herbal teas, juices (especially with fruits and vegetables that have high water content).

7. If you cannot digest milk or feel heavy after drinking it, ensure you always warm it (this is important for everybody) and dilute it by adding ginger and cardamom.

8. Ayurveda says ghee is vital to good health, increases strength of the body, and calms the mind. I recommend three to five tea-spoons a day.

9. Chew your food to mix digestive enzymes with it. This is one of the reasons why silence is often advocated when eating, to focus on the food.

10. Add ginger or black pepper to your meal, or sip ginger tea after meals to stimulate digestion.

11. Chew on fennel seeds after your meal.

12. Keep tea and coffee moderate, as excess caffeine can create toxins.

Make Cleansing Part of Your Routine

I've been cleansing regularly for decades and inherently I know when it is time to do it. Sometimes, I override this innate calling to cleanse, but then I usually experience the consequences. When I am cleansing, I feel like a blank canvas on which I can paint anything with my life. All the colors in the palate are available to me at my choosing. It's the most empowering, wonderful, light feeling. I feel powerful when I cleanse, and I've worked with so many women who feel empowered by cleansing, too.

When I cleanse, I have more radiance. There is more spark in my being. My eyes shine. When I'm cleansing, people are usually drawn to my eyes and will ask what I am doing because they see something so alive and they want it, too!

I recently prepared myself for my role as teaching assistant in an intensive teacher training program in India. I did a seven-day mung soup cleanse with a group of women from The Radiant Woman community. As you well know, life can become even more hectic and full when preparing to be away from home for an extended amount of time. My intention for the cleanse was to clear the clutter and accumulation and align myself as best I could to be of service: light, clear, and present. During the training, a virus stormed through the group. Teachers and students became really ill with fever, aches, pains, headache, cough, diarrhea... the full gamut of viral symptoms. The classroom was like a hospital ward with masks, and beds on the floor. Without wearing a mask, and consciously pulling back on the chai, I did not become ill. I attribute this in significant part to doing a mung cleanse. My gut was not a ripe host for the virus. The nasty little sucker would have passed through me like everyone else, but my gut was not an inviting home for it to settle in because I'd cleaned it up. My immune integrity was solid from the immediate benefits of cleansing to bolster digestion and metabolic processes.

Regular cleansing is a great panacea to remove fatigue. It really does bestow the gift of vitality. When I cleanse, my sleep becomes more refreshing, deeper. The quality of my dreams changes. My gut and body become lighter. I observe a more steadfast energy throughout the day without peaks and troughs. Meditation is better. My mind is more focused, still, with better mental clarity. I feel more connected to myself and my family. I can see bigger pictures, broader vistas. There is a greater mental flexibility, the grip loosens, and there is more ease to flow with life. There is renewal.

I was doing a three-day recalibrate cleanse with a group in my community. One woman shared that her husband did not believe in what she was doing but decided to join in eating what she was eating because she was chief cook and that's all there was prepared. It was a whole green mung soup cleanse. He immediately felt better and had more refreshing sleep. He did not get up during the night for the first time in years. He was astounded to awake without the chronic stiffness and pain in his feet that he usually experienced each morning.

He still did not believe in the benefits of the cleanse with the mung soup ... it was pure coincidence and a miracle that his feet were pain free!

Mung soup is a mono-food fast and this is the most effective way to reduce inflammation anywhere in the body, from the finest to grossest of channels.

Mung Bean Soup

In Ayurveda, the million-dollar food and way to cleanse the tissues of accumulation is whole green mung bean soup. Mung is light and easy to digest. It is a clever food because it has the capacity to convert metabolic sludge into energy in the body. Mung gives the body the capacity to do what it must do while our organs of digestion rest and we have the opportunity to recalibrate.

Some foods are tri-dośic, which means that they are generally suitable and nourishing for everybody and not aggravating for anybody. Mung soup, when prepared a certain way, is one such food. Being easily digestible, mung soup rests the load of the digestive organs. It allows them to reorganize, recalibrate, and simply operate more efficiently. This means you use your food more wisely and it goes where it needs to go in the body. It does not remain where it ought not, creating residual sludge and blockage (aam).

Mung soup stabilizes you. When this food is eaten regularly, blood sugar stabilizes, and the dośas, which govern all processes in the body, stabilize. Mung soup encourages mobilization of blockages, which allows excess accumulation of the dośas to be eradicated via the gut and organs of elimination. It cleans up your inner landscape, especially the channels of your mind. Hallelujah! How good is that?

There are ways to prepare mung soup that render it more easily digestible.

Being a hard, little legume, it must be cooked to the point of being completely homogenized. That means it loses its individual identity. If you eat it hard, then you will get gas and perhaps bloating or heaviness. One effective way to prepare mung is to soak it for a few hours or even overnight, in some water, before cooking (do not cook sprouted mung—that's a completely different taste and effect).

There are many different ways you can prepare mung soup, including, as is so commonly asked, adding vegetables to the pot. When using this food to eliminate or cleanse, this is the most *sāttvic*, or purest, way for optimal cleansing benefits.

Occasionally, people have a complete aversion to mung soup. For these people, I recommend cleansing with a vegetable broth soup, without using tomato, potato, or cabbage. You can use pumpkin, zucchini, squash, spinach, chard (silver beet), broccoli, celery, and sweet potato. The soup is more broth-like and not pureed or creamed. Additionally, some people with very sensitive digestion and food allergies experience bloating and discomfort when eating mung soup. In such instances, I recommend following the recipe in appendix C, strictly as given, including full soaking, homogenizing, and adding asafetida and spices. Take more of the broth and less of the bean on a cleansing day. Gradually adjust as the digestion strengthens and creates a healthy inner boundary to be able to tolerate and digest more efficiently.

Cleansing with Mung

The one-day cleanse is a gentle cleanse and suitable for everybody. You can do it regularly.

Just as many people in many cultures fast one day a week, you can do a mung fast one day a week for wellness and good digestive health. Generally, I do not encourage liquid-only fasts with water or juice in Ayurveda. Under supervision or upon a practitioner's recommendation, this may be prescribed in some situations. However, usually I encourage a mono-food fast with mung soup or vegetable soup.

To do a one-day mung fast, weekly, fortnightly, or monthly you simply eat mung soup for all meals and in-between. Do not go hungry, and eat regularly throughout the day, but only this food. When fasting with mung soup, the soup is prepared with more broth, like dal but with a thicker consistency. Make enough soup so that you can eat as much as you need to satisfy you and maintain your stamina throughout the day. If you leave the house, make sure you bring a thermos of the soup. If you are hungry between meals, have a cup of the soup, even just the broth.

You can sip on ginger tea throughout the day or drink a metabolic tea blend of ginger, cumin, and coriander. Drinking hot water after a meal aids the digestive processes and reduces the accumulation of aam. Sipping hot water throughout the day helps to reduce vata. This is especially helpful if you have to talk a lot, which increases vata.

When you cleanse with mung soup, do not eat meat, dairy, or flour. These foods have heavy, building, and sticky qualities, counteracting the eliminating and cleansing action of the mung soup.

If you've eaten a particularly heavy meal, or if you are going to, then you can do a mung soup cleanse for a day or even half a day. This will help your body fully digest your last meal as well as prepare you to be able to digest the heavy food coming your way.

If you wish to go deeper, then prepare yourself and do a three-day mung soup cleanse. Start the day with one teaspoon of ghee in hot water. In the evening before bed, take one teaspoon of castor oil or vaca oil, followed with ginger tea if you wish. Vaca oil is a medicated castor oil with bitter herbs that have a scraping effect on the tissues and any accumulation in them.

A three-day cleanse will go deeper and mobilize more internally, so it is better to plan and prepare so that you can meet it without too much tension or resistance. If your life is too busy to accommodate the cleanse with ease, for example, if you're relocating or getting married, then it is not a good time to do the cleanse.

There is a seven-day radiance mung cleanse (see appendix A) and some even do a maha thirteen-day mung cleanse. However, I recommend that these longer cleanses be done with the supervision of an Ayurvedic practitioner.

When doing a mung soup cleanse, you will still have good energy to do all your daily tasks and moderate exercise. If you're doing a seven-day or longer cleanse and you are used to eating meat regularly, you may feel less physical strength. This is one of the aspects that you will need to include in your planning and preparation.

Also, the longer the cleanse, the more vulnerable you will be when finishing it. Your digestion is sensitized, and so you introduce foods gradually and moderately on coming out of a cleanse. Even after a one-day cleanse, a huge steak and chips as your first meal would be hard to digest. Not only is your gut tissue cleaner and more sensitive, but your mental channels are cleaner, more open and sensitive to all the impressions and experiences you take in.

Should You Fast?

When cleansing Ayurvedically, it is not encouraged to fast without food, unless under particular circumstances with the supervision of an experienced practitioner. I recommend fasting without food only under supervision, for a day or two at most, with ginger tea.

When you fast, a space is created in the body. If this space is not managed correctly, it will fill up with vata, which will travel upward into the mental channels, which will fill up with too much air element. This makes people ungrounded and, for some, they can manage it. However, for many it is too much, and they become destabilized. I've often had to manage and support people who have overenthusiastically fasted and feel "high" on the extra gases and air in the mental channels, a "heady" feeling.

One patient presented to me with insomnia and lots of irritability and inner agitation. She felt that life was shortchanging her. She was feeling like a victim. She did not like thinking and feeling this way and desperately wanted good sleep. This woman was also in the habit of fasting without food one day every week.

Her pulse had too much vata, which was creating problems not only in her joints, but also in her mental channels. It was making her feel oversensitive, overreactive.

Her more subtle bodies, which in anthroposophical medicine are known as the astral (or feelings) body and ego organization or "I," were unable to loosen from her life organization and physical body as they do each night in a healthy sleep. These subtle body forces of the astral feeling body and "I" are strongly carried and embodied in the force of vata. They're aggravated when vata is disturbed and needs pacifying and vice versa.

To replace her fast, we introduced a mono-food day, with either mung soup or vegetable soup, on a weekly basis. For this woman, with her particular constitution, it was not encouraged to cleanse or fast without food (unless she had a fever).

Final Thoughts on Cleansing

Cleansing keeps clear the channels and tissues of our mind, body, and emotional life. It keeps us that bit more connected to experiencing a purposeful life. It removes stress from our body. Some accumulations get carted away while we sleep, some through our exhalation, some through our elimination, and some literally perspired or flushed away. Occasionally, you can feel discomfort as the very cells in which you have held this accumulation, deep in storage, are opened and things are mobilized back into circulation. You can experience this discomfort with resistance, fear, restlessness, and uncertainty. This is why we prepare ourselves to cleanse in a way that is conducive to our best experience.

Your inherent blueprint remains as is destined. However, you have a greater experience of being your best possible self, emphasizing and fully utilizing your gifts, when cleaning the inner pathways.

By bringing yourself back into your center, when cleansing you are emphasizing your strengths and not constantly feeding the weaker aspects of yourself.

In this process, you bolster your digestive fire, rekindle your agni. The fire pit is cleaned and there is space again to fan the flames of your fuel. As a woman, your inner rhythms are reestablished, metabolic processes improved and made more efficient. Your hormones become more aligned. Your aggravated excesses become more pacified and you become more connected to your heart.

Thus, to cleanse is a great gesture of self-compassion. When cleansing, you are receiving empathy from yourself. And thus, filling your cups, you can have more empathy for others. In essence cleansing brings balance back into your life.

CHAPTER 12

Deep Nourishment

· · · · · · · · · · · · ·

NOURISHMENT, IN TERMS of food, is something that can benefit or hinder your whole development as a human being. Nourishment feeds you so that you may grow and thrive. It supports you and allows you to live your life purposefully.

Deep nourishment means feeding your essential nature as you mature and evolve. That means looking at nourishment for your tissues, organs, and cycles as a woman, including your uterine health. It also means nourishing your spirit. Contemplate how the life forces change and transform all your seasons and thresholds, for refined growth and purpose.

When I write about food, when I prescribe or recommend eating or avoiding certain foods, I am making general recommendations based on holistic principles that will, according to Ayurveda, benefit your entire development as a human being.

However, philosophically, whether you eat meat, drink alcohol, or smoke cigarettes, it is not for me to say what is right or wrong for you and the evolution of your humanness. My task is to explain how foods and other substances act and their nutritional effect in terms of your vitality. Of course, what you do with this information is completely your prerogative. Nobody else can choose for you. Even when I prescribe clinically, a person has to choose to receive and take responsibility for the remedy. You could say that nourishment is a task of free will. It cannot be forced upon you. I can only guide you to discern what you need to nourish yourself.

What is nourishing for me may not be nourishing for you and vice versa, based on our individual circumstances at this moment in life, constitutionally or demographically.

My intention is to impart principles and guidelines that you can instinctively recognize and then determine the right action and nourishment for you at this time. When I write of nutritional substance, in essence I am writing about something that not only supports your physical and mental wellness but benefits your spiritual development, too.

In the modern world, which puts so much emphasis on the external, nutrition is viewed also in such light. To be whole and complete, as you are, the approach needs to be spiritually and scientifically based. All nutrition, to me, needs to be holistic. It must consider the internal as well as the external—the rich inner life, the soul life, and how the substance nourishes this aspect of you.

How does the nourishing substance affect the innermost aspect of you and your relationship with other human beings, animals, and plants?

We know that nourishment keeps us alive. We know that when it is gone, the physical elements decay. So we nourish both seen and unseen parts of ourselves.

Inner flexibility, the ability to flow with life, gives the very foundation and pillar for any nutritional problem. Hold this thought and contemplate a deficiency in certain nutrients. What is really lacking? Can a supplement truly fix a problem? Albeit our soils are depleted and deficient in certain minerals, nutrients, and amino acids that we may require for good processes and health. But nutrition composes a bigger image than the physical substance of the food itself. It is true that some diets, particularly vegan or vegetarian, may be lacking in certain minerals and nutrients. However, there is more to the whole picture of nutrients than the composition of food—humans also require nourishing food for soul development.

Our bodily tissues, the dhātus, are involved in the total health and whole function of the organism. Each dhātu in itself has a specific sphere of functionality and purpose. These tissues are nourished by particular foods, how we process with the right warmth, and digest, secrete, or maintain material.

The kind of nourishment we take in, digest, refine, and pass along is what feeds the dhātu. It will take and extract what it needs to nourish itself for optimal functionality and pass along to the next digestive fire to feed that dhātu.

Then we have our organs, which have different governing forces. In addition, our organs are affected by planetary influences and corresponding metals that influence each organ of the body. And, just as they have governing forces, they have different physical qualities that affect the human body. They have different tasks and they relate to certain qualities of feelings. For example, kidneys relate to the feelings of fear. The liver relates to our discernment, discrimination, and joy. Our spleen relates to the underlying digestive rhythms of everything we take in.

Our organs and how we nourish them are of great importance.

We nourish also with cycles. This means eating seasonal foods that nourish the inner seasonal conditions of our being. In summertime, for example, the elements of warmth are greater, so we eat more cooling and pacifying foods. In winter, when the elements are cooler and damper, we eat more warming, unctuous, and stimulating foods. Eating in this way is how we nourish our seasonal cycles.

Nourishment not only comes through the food we eat but through our relationship to it. To our relationship to ourselves, one another, our life's purpose, our life's work, the very earth, and the elements that produce the food. Nourishment comes from having purpose and meaning in life, from being connected to our self. This is deep nourishment. It comes from being in touch with our feelings and our needs. It comes not only from giving but from receiving. Nourishment is thus reciprocal.

The nourishment of self-love is possibly the most potent nourishment we can give ourselves. As women, we are masters at giving love to others but not always so great at giving ourselves the nourishment of self-love.

An important nourishment we take in is cosmic nourishment, a nourishment that is not possible to source in the earthly realm. We absorb, through our inhalation and skin, the tiniest particles of cosmic nourishment that are showering down and subtly being ingested regularly. When we sleep, we receive this cosmic nourishment.

As I sat on the river stones and became absorbed in the
beauty and mighty sounds of the of the river I heard her speak.
O woman, be sure you are soft and at ease. For a
moment simply leaving the demands and burdens of your day,
your stories, your life, be present to the miracle you are.
Gift this to your divine essence. The reverberating sound of your
heart song. The sound that resonates so subtly and tenderly
awaits your nourishment. The nourishment that feeds your heart
center. The nourishment of your womanhood.

Our plants ingest this cosmic nourishment too, particularly plants that are grown biodynamically. This is why biodynamic food possesses a particular quality of nourishment that cannot be found in any other method of food growing. This kind of nourishment, while invisible to the human eye, is the most nutrient-dense nourishment we can receive.

According to Ayurveda, uterine health is the seat of a woman's creativity. How, then, do we nourish uterine health as the seat of women's good health and of her creative expression? Creative expression is a very important, nourishing substance. This is the capacity to express oneself creatively. You have innate and diverse ways of doing this, big or small. We have the intrinsic capacity to create, and it is vital for our nourishment that we do so. Of course, we also have the infinite capacity to create life.

It is important to creatively express yourself throughout your life. Whatever lights you up: dance, cook, sing, sew, knit, garden, pull weeds, make daisy chains, draw, journal, paint, sculpt with clay, paint murals on the kitchen cupboards. The possibilities are endless. Creative expression is the way you admire the beauty in nature and how nature moves through you. You can read poetry. You can write poetry. It's in the way you hang the clothing on the line, butter your toast, and even slice your bread. The point is that it is important to do and acknowledge that you are expressing yourself freely from pure imagination, in a way that brings you freedom, beauty, and joy. To understand and listen to your feelings and needs, allow yourself to resonate with this thread of creative expression as it pulsates within you.

A great way to express yourself creatively is through your written words. Sit for guidance or meditation and then write… it's a beautiful way for the divine creative expression of words to flow through you.

I am everywhere, infusing everything.
To find me,
become absorbed in intense experience.
Go all the way.
Be drenched in the energies of life.

Enter the world beyond separation.
The light of a candle reveals a room.
The rays of the sun reveal the world.
So does the divine feminine
Illumine the way to me.

BANTER VERSE 21, *THE RADIANCE SUTRAS*

III

Stages
of Life

CHAPTER 13

Childhood, the Formative Growth Years, and Reproduction

. . . .

AYURVEDA TEACHES US that there are three phases of a person's life. These phases each see a dominance of one of the governing dośas. That is why we call the phases "the kapha phase," "the pitta phase," and "the vata phase."

From birth to sixteen years of age is the kapha phase of life. The cohesion and structure of our physical architecture is put in place. The temple of our spirit is constructed by the inherent design and forces of nature so that we may do our life's work on Earth. How cool is that? Simultaneously, constant inner processes are being created, formed, and developed, which requires incredible building, nourishing, lubricating, unctuous forces to grow optimally.

It makes sense that in this phase of life our earth and water forces are greater, for building and nourishing. It is a phase of growth, and kapha forces are growth forces.

Relating to phlegm and mucus, our kapha years are also our snot years! This is why young children, particularly up to the age of seven to nine, can be little walking snot units. As there is more kapha generally, there can be a tendency for more congestion, upper respiratory tract infections, overproduction of mucus, tonsillitis, cold, cough, throat, ear infections, and childhood asthma. Take comfort, dear ones, this is a brief moment in a person's biography and also not a given for each child. Individual constitutions determine whether there is excess of kapha.

This, too, is why children need more sleep as discussed in greater detail in chapter 9. The growth forces are so great that the inertia and heaviness of this phase commands greater periods of rest in order to maintain balance. Sleep is necessary to support enormous growth. Imagine the growth forces in a newborn baby. We can all see when growth is happening in children. There are growth spurts, and after a long deep sleep, a child seems to have developed inwardly and outwardly before our very eyes. It is wondrous to behold and reflect upon.

Foods are eaten that encourage growth and production of tissue. Nourishing, hearty, building foods like whole wheat, slow-cooked meats, whole milk, sweet melons, basmati rice, almonds, pistachios, dates, root vegetables, butter, and ghee.

Children simply embody all the kapha attributes of generosity, abundance, love, and nourishment. It oozes from their very being. It is the essence of who they are. And, just like the flip side of kapha attributes, they can be possessive and greedy!

The kapha phase of life creates a physical structure that is well nourished and supports a woman in her reproductive years. The good juices and tissues are grown in readiness to be able to create and birth, to nourish through mothering just like Mother Earth, and to keep enough to stay inwardly nourished and well.

Whether or not a woman births children, it is still important to nourish these tissues and the kapha so that she can birth well any creative process or expression undertaken in life. The good juices and tissues here foster good creative expression.

This phase is one of form and abundance, so we need to nourish well in ways that establish foundations for life. Rhythms and the imitation of parents, family, and educators of the child, are key here, along with good nourishment and sleep as a young girl grows.

Having a rhythm to life is essential because this lends a harmony that creates balance in our life, which is vital for balance in hormonal health. We cannot have one without the other.

The Dynamic Fertile Years and Woman's Sacred Rhythm of Menstrual Cycles

At her first period a girl meets her wisdom.
Through her menstruating years she practices her wisdom.
At menopause she becomes her wisdom.
NATIVE AMERICAN SAYING

Becoming wisdom means embodying wisdom. To embody wisdom, however, your vata dośa must be balanced. It is simply not possible to embody your wisdom unless this vata is pacified.

The pitta phase of life comprise the reproductive years. A young woman's digestion is key to wellness here as digestion governs the immune integrity, emotional intelligence, and vitality that a girl must have much to navigate the tumultuous passage of teenage years. You need good, nourishing substance to hold you in the vast phase of reproductive years, especially to keep the mental channels pacified as a young girl embarks upon this major navigation of meeting herself as a woman.

Metabolic processes and reproductive hormones depend on good digestive health for flow and optimal health in this pitta phase of life. It is here that the impressions, experiences, and demands of life are at their greatest. We are talking from teen years to the cessation of the cycle. That's a lot of living, and an enormous amount of vitality, discrimination, and decision making. Wow. I reflect briefly on my life since my first menstrual cycle on my thirteenth birthday, and it's been mammoth and full beyond anything I could have imagined.

Menstrual Cycle

Uterine health is the seat of a woman's good health, and the source of your womanhood. It is the seat of your creative health. Whether you wish to have children or not it is vital to have good endocrine and uterine health.

A healthy menstrual cycle is typically twenty-eight days beginning at the first day of bleeding. It is three to five days in duration, not too light and not too heavy. It comes without pain, discomfort, bloating and fluid retention, extreme fatigue, headache, nausea, irritability, breast tenderness, or emotional extremes. These are all signs of a hormonal imbalance.

We are purpose-filled beings. There is a divine purpose and plan for each of us. We are connected to our children, parents, siblings, friends, community, and all beings on Earth. If we are not connected to ourselves, our innate rhythms, then what are we teaching our children? We have a duty to ourselves, to our daughters, families, and communities to pay attention to our rhythms and cycles.

As women, this is self-love in action and it is shaping our future. It is part of woman's capacity to meet and heal the challenges we face in our modern world. When we connect to the wisdom of our cycle, we remember great insight and understanding of life's mysteries.

Nourishing and harmonizing your inner rhythms comes more easily to some than to others for a plethora of reasons. But whether it comes naturally to you or not, please be vigilant and disciplined to nourish your daily needs, and experience your best possible life, particularly in the second half of your life from menopause and after. Once you lose your vitality, it becomes increasingly difficult to build up again. Your vitality is a treasure to be guarded with great vigilance and vigor.

Women, you have a duty to give yourselves permission to pull back and do less, be more and to take more rest. Nobody else can give you this permission. If you do not give it to yourself, learning to take rest and repose, how can our daughters imitate good nourishing patterns and establish habits for wellness for their own hormonal health and lives? You do not have to be a mother to have this sacred duty. All daughters imitate you as a woman. You are connected to the influence of every woman and daughter on this planet. Yes, it may be subtle, but it is true. There is a golden thread that binds us all together and you cannot be the best version of yourself until every other woman is the best version of herself. You are the teachers. You have to teach our daughters. The world needs you to teach one another and our daughters. It is time to step fully into this, dear one. It is your time to honor your precious life as a woman. You can absolutely be an Ayurvedic woman.

During our menstrual cycle, we need to eat gentle foods and exercise gently, appropriately for this precious time where we are wide open and vulnerable. Subtle channels are open as we eliminate and bleed. Digestion is weaker as digestive energy is directed toward our womb and the menstruation processes. Emotions are heightened naturally and we have less physical energy. We support this process in a healthy way when we rest more and say no to what does not serve us at the time of bleeding.

Honor those you love most by honoring yourself and your cycle. Love your cycle. This is loving the essence of who you are as woman. If you cannot love it, then get help to balance your cycle so you can fall in love with yourself.

Many women do not slow or adjust their pace at all during a menstrual cycle. For some women, it is even considered an inconvenience, a pest, and synthetic hormones or devices are implanted so they do not bleed at all. It is inconceivable to block such an inherent part of your nature so that you can continue to live in a way that is removed from your feminine way. Of course, you can choose to do this. If it is your preference, then so be it. However, nature does have laws that are intrinsically related to your inner nature. If you choose to live against the laws of nature, you will not win. You cannot take on nature and win. I say pick your fights wisely, dear woman!

I absolutely understand why many women seek the support of synthetic hormones. However, they are not a long-term solution to hormonal disturbances. When you are in crisis, just as it takes a village to raise a child, it takes a multidisciplinary team of holistic health practitioners and therapists to truly meet and treat the health crisis. This is the kind of assistance I encourage you to seek if you have a chronic health challenge and are being recommended synthetic hormones as a "solution." In an interview with me, Dr. Claudia Welch shared that under no circumstance would she recommend synthetic hormones. Where absolutely necessary, for example, a woman going into menopause with compromised bone density, osteopenia, or osteoporosis, may require a bioidentical hormone but not a synthetic one.

I recommend you read *Balance Your Hormones, Balance Your Life* by Dr. Claudia Welch. It comprehensively describes and explains synthetic hormones and the hormonal processes of a woman. It's an easy read and great resource to have.

Many women push hard and do not adjust their exercise routines and training during menstruation, running marathons, triathlons, and sometimes pushing their bodies so hard that their menstrual cycle cannot come. What is nature telling us in such extremes?

Learning to be able to sit with yourself and be in your own company without distraction at the time of bleeding is deeply nourishing and connecting. The veils are thin at menstruation and you get knowledgeable, beautiful insight into yourself.

Practicing wisdom during menarche years means using the opportunity to learn about who you are through your cycles and nature. It is a time to reflect, observe, and learn about yourself, preparing you for the second half of your life. The health established in the menarche years is what creates the foundation of wellness at this time. It absolutely affects your experience at the cessation of menses including physical energy, purpose, enthusiasm, and ease as aging forces prevail.

Menstrual Discomfort

Our blood carries life force and consciousness. When we bleed, we cleanse what we no longer need; however, if we bleed too much, we lose too much vital life force and lose a grip on this consciousness. It must be balanced. Some will always bleed more or less than others. Of course, this is healthy and fine, but how do we know what is a "healthy" range and what is imbalance?

Many difficulties women commonly experience during their menstrual cycle are due to too much vata, pitta, and inflammation of the reproductive channels and organs. The subtle channels, tissues, and organs of our reproductive system fill with air and swelling (gas and fluid). These create varying levels of discomfort within a woman's menstrual cycle, including painful and scanty menstruation, excessive bleeding, foul-smelling blood, mid-cycle bleeding, headaches, nausea, anxiety, irritation, depression, painful ovulation, endometriosis, fibroids, polycystic ovaries, and backache.

Up to one third of women in Australia regularly use anti-inflammatory medication to relieve dysmenorrhea. Many women experience intense, debilitating pain and discomfort and know no other effective way to manage the pain. This can go on for years, even decades, and for some women their entire menarche years. It can be so extreme that some women choose to have their reproductive organs physically removed.

Many women take pain relievers during their menstrual cycle to avoid the inconvenience their discomfort presents. That means not taking rest or slowing down but putting on a bandage and fulfilling obligations as scheduled. The show must go on! I totally get it, but if you have to take pain relief to manage your menstrual cycle to be able to keep functioning at your optimum, then you are forcing against your nature and there will be consequences. The thing is, we don't know what we don't know, and if you think your discomfort is a "normal" part of your cycle, then it becomes your normal.

But a recent study, published in April 2018, in an article in *American Journal Obstetrics & Gynecology* has shown that in up to 20 percent of women, anti-inflammatory drugs do not even alleviate their menstrual pain.

I have seen a thousand times the effectiveness of Ayurvedic treatment with all of the above menstrual disorders and female health challenges. The treatments will usually focus on eliminating excess accumulation of vata and pitta from the lower abdomen and removing swelling, bulkiness, and inflammation.

As aam blocks the channels of the reproductive system and channels of elimination and circulation, it also aggravates the vata and pitta. Thus, it's necessary to focus on reducing accumulation in the tissues, too.

If you experience any menstrual discomfort, it's recommended that you avoid eating sour and fermented foods, including the following: tomatoes, yogurt, lemon, heavy beans (kidney beans, lima beans, and chickpeas).

Mandy, age thirty-six, came to one of my menstrual health workshops many years ago. She had struggled with her menstrual cycle for twenty years. It was heavy; she had regular cramping, backache, a heavy "dragging-down" feeling and leg tiredness every month. After attending my workshop, she stopped eating sour and fermented foods. Just by avoiding these foods, particularly tomatoes (cooked and fresh) and yogurt (she had been it eating daily for breakfast), she experienced no cramping or pain with her next menstruation. She continued, and after four months, the heaviness of her bleeding had reduced, she was without menstrual discomfort, and she had more life energy.

This example illustrates how the bulkiness and inflammation were reduced when Mandy eliminated the sour foods that were aggravating her pitta, leading to metabolic heat and retention of fluid.

Pregnancy

Thank you for honoring yourself in pregnancy, and for choosing to learn more about your body and being in a deeper, richer way from the perspective of Ayurveda. Lord Dhanvantari, the deity of Ayurveda, would be delighted, I'm sure!

There can be a romantic notion of how pregnancy will be. This is purely an imaginative picture and so often conceptual only. Sometimes, for a plethora of reasons, pregnancy is not what you thought it would or could possibly be.

The truth is that pregnancy can be tough and really hard work because of your life circumstances making the timing awkward. You may have conceived when depleted, tired, and fatigued by life challenges, including monetary, relationship, housing, climatic, political, and social reasons. It may be that you just feel like crap and are experiencing an unearthly fatigue that renders you horizontal on the sofa, unable to will yourself upright to walk to the sink to wash the dirty dishes. You may feel particularly nauseous. You may feel heavy, like you are dragging a chain, with nagging aches and pains. You could be constantly running, running, running, and there is no space for you to be barefoot, picking flowers, and celebrating with the world, "Hooray, I'm pregnant!"

Pregnancy can be a daunting time for many women. Some women choose a cesarean because it is too scary to truly contemplate giving birth. Other women have a plan to birth without intervention, at home or in the hospital. There are so many different ways you can choose how you ideally wish to birth. Your plan may not play out the way that you had visualized it would. And, when this occurs, how do you meet it? How do you respond and flow with the unforeseen birth circumstances?

From an Ayurvedic perspective, when you bring your doṣas into alignment as much as you possibly can, you are able to respond with awareness to whatever presents. In this awareness, you can choose your response to your experiences. It's ultimately okay, because you can respond to your birth situation and rise to meet it. This is your innate capacity as a woman. Nothing is given to you that is greater than you. It's not less than you. You are not better than any challenge that presents, but it is not greater than you either. When you are aligned, you can respond instead of purely reacting to whatever scenario you are called to face.

Of course, there are things you can do to support and change how you are feeling, not only physically but mentally and emotionally, too. There are things that you can tweak. They can be really small and simple things, such as adjusting the foods that you eat, taking simple home remedies, or changing daily lifestyle practices. These tweaks nourish your internal rhythms and elements that are constantly dancing and playing out to change your experience of pregnancy from mediocre to extraordinary!

The five elements, according to Ayurveda, are also responsible for the growth and development of the fetus. The air element, vāyu, is what enables the division of cells in pregnancy. Fire, agni, enables digestion and metabolism, metabolic processes of the cells as they divide and grow. Water, jala, is the moisture. The element of earth, pṛthvī, gives compactness and stability to the fetus. Space, ākāśa, provides the environment in which the fetus can grow.

Elementally, it is a dance of creation as the child grows within the womb.

Ayurvedically, the focus on diet in pregnancy is purely and primarily around giving nourishment, strength, and stability to the mother. The baby is fine and receives all his or her needs when the mother has all her nourishment.

Babies are clever. They take the nourishment that they need. It's just so important to keep giving deep nourishment to yourself so that you don't go into a deficit, which can show up years later. Hence, it's all about deeply nourishing yourself, giving yourself strength and stability from the subtle to the grossest aspects of you, all your tissues and being.

This emphasis on diet in pregnancy gives your pelvic organs all the inherent strength, stability, and nourishment that they need. It gives the tissues the inherent strength that they need. It gives the skin the inherent strength that it needs to do its work. Ultimately, that translates as an easier delivery.

Ayurveda says that when a woman has abnormal cravings throughout pregnancy, it is something to be noted. In pregnancy, craving indicates an innate yearning for something that needs to be nourished within the mother. The mother needs something in the substance that she craves. At other times, craving a particular food or taste may be feeding an imbalance or aggravated dominant doṣa.

In Ayurveda, it is said to never suppress a natural urge, and this is particularly true in pregnancy. Especially, never suppress the urges of peeing, pooping, farting, or burping. To illustrate, let's look at urinating. Apāna vāyu is the major state of movement down through your abdominal cavity, urinary tract, and organs, as well as through the reproductive organs. Since it is responsible for movement, and because it is composed of air, it is very unstable and moves erratically. If it wants to move in a certain direction, and you ignore it and don't move it immediately, the air that is the driving force behind that impulse goes to places it ought not to go. Not blocking the flow and release is important advice for everyone in all phases of life, but particularly in pregnancy, as it's all about easing delivery and supporting the birth passage of a soul into this earthly life.

Post-pregnancy, take care that there is no air in the uterine cavity and no extra air in the tissues. This air can show up as backache, hip pain, difficulty with menstrual cycles, menstrual discomfort, pain, and inflammation. It can even result in emotional and mental instability because too much air moves upward and impacts vata in the region of your emotions and mental channels.

The first trimester is all about strengthening fetal development so that the uterus will hold on tight. We know that physiologically it is a vulnerable time, but according to Ayurveda it's also a spiritually vulnerable time. The pregnant woman has to nourish herself so that the spiritual connection with the fetus can also be held.

You can use certain home remedies to support this connection. In the first and second month, you can take between three to five teaspoons of ghee daily. In the first few months of pregnancy there is so much vata dominance. The cells are dividing and multiplying at such a rapid rate, which creates lots of movement that the ghee pacifies. The metabolic processes, the pitta, are also pacified by the ghee. Ghee just makes thing flow the way they ought to flow. It is very nourishing to have ghee at all times but particularly in the first and second months of your pregnancy.

Eat lots of zucchini, which is very important at this time. Another very supportive remedy is white pumpkin juice. This juice is good for all kinds of conditions and particularly for mothers in the first trimester. In Australia and New Zealand, we do not have access to white pumpkin for its juice. The closest food with similar properties that we have access to is zucchini, for its cooling, pacifying, building, and nourishing qualities. It's better to eat it cooked. Although it's not very appetizing juiced alone, you can add zucchini or white pumpkin to other vegetable and fruit juices.

Combined with apple and carrot, it's a tasty and very supportive juice.

During pregnancy, your constitution influences and shapes the constitution of your baby. Whatever you are more dominant in, whether vata, pitta, or kapha, your child inherits these elements. It's perfect, as you have been chosen to be the mother of this particular soul!

The baby also has a constitutional blueprint and dominance of these governing forces. Your body not only has to metabolize and process for you, it's also processing for the baby and influenced by the baby's metabolic processes. If you have lots of vata, lots of gas and wind, and the baby has existed in that, yours is going to be more aggravated. That's really important, Ayurvedically, especially in the first trimester, because that downward movement (apāna vāyu) can affect whether or not the pregnancy is viable. It affects the inherent strength of your tissues' elasticity, malleability, and flexibility.

It's similar with pitta, which is typically experienced in the first trimester, and for some women throughout the whole pregnancy, as nausea and headaches.

I had a woman come and see me clinically a few years ago. It was her second pregnancy. Her first pregnancy had been really uncomfortable the whole time. It was such a relief to give birth because she was nauseous and vomiting throughout the pregnancy. She would have headaches. She wasn't feeling the shiny glow of pregnancy. She was suffering, and her mantra was "When is it going to be over?"

Each day of pregnancy was really hard work for her. And, here she was, pregnant again. The joy of being pregnant was totally overshadowed by the thought, "This is going to be really hard work and I just don't know if I am going to be up for it."

Already, it was difficult for her to come see me in clinic because her nausea was just so great. She couldn't keep anything down. We simply worked with her diet. She had so much heat in her body that we tweaked a few things to alleviate the heat, to pacify and cool her down. We removed sour foods and pungent, heating foods, of which she was eating a lot. We added ghee to her diet. She also took powder of coral, which is very pacifying. The coral and also turmeric helped with the nausea.

Things really turned around for her. At six to seven months of pregnancy she was sitting in the clinic and said, "I am just loving it. I am loving being pregnant."

I said, "Listen to you! Bravo!"

She was able to really enjoy her pregnancy, but that wouldn't have been the case had she kept heading down the same path. She was doing things nutritionally that were very good for her, but she didn't understand that she had a lot of heat, a lot of pitta, and her metabolic processes combined with those of the baby were too much. They needed to be pacified and cooled. She birthed another magnificent, fiery little redhead. Hence, dear ones, there are things that can be done for nausea, no matter how great it is.

In the third to fourth month of pregnancy, the fetal heartbeat appears and the mother is termed *hṛidaya*, which means one who has two hearts. You can feel that in the pulse—the heart of the baby as well as the heart of the mother; it is quite beautiful.

Two weeks before delivery, at about thirty-eight weeks of pregnancy, apāna vāyu starts to move very differently, mobilizing. That time is all about helping that vata move in the right direction, downward, to facilitate an easy delivery. At this point, you can take a teaspoon of castor oil each night before bed.

I know a woman who came to full term and wanted to birth "now" and just get it out of the way to get on with things. (I cannot imagine what things would be more important at such a time....) She became impatient and took lots of castor oil and went into distress. She birthed very quickly, too quickly. It was traumatic for her and the baby. Taking too much castor oil (even just two teaspoons) will have a purgative effect and force downward-moving vāyu and the birthing process. One teaspoon will make sure that vata is pacified and moving in the right direction.

Ayurveda and yoga are sister sciences. One leads, loops around, and merges with the other. They lead a woman into herself, to a deeper understanding of herself. Yoga means "to yoke," so you can more fully understand and touch the infinite greatness of who you are, what your experiences in life are, and why you have them. Pregnancy is such a divine and perfect time to explore this aspect of yourself as a woman.

If not doing so already, I encourage pregnant women to start chanting *auṁ* because it's not only a primordial sound of which all sound was born in the universe, but it has a resonance. That resonance works within your body. When I chant my auṁ, I like to think of that resonance finely tuning my compass. I think each of us has an internal compass and it guides us in life. If you've used a compass, they are pretty delicate. Their movement is so fine that it's important to keep it as accurate as possible because it carries a consciousness within us. That is what connects us to the experience of who we are.

Yoga *āsana* practice in pregnancy supports and strengthens, creates inner spaciousness and prepares all aspects of woman to facilitate an easeful delivery. It supports the recovery and renewal of woman post-delivery.

Just as gestation takes forty weeks, it takes an equal amount of time for the mother's renewal post-delivery. The mother has the tissue and sensitivity of the delicate newborn. She is to be handled with tenderness and care. Women need the support of family, friends, and community after birthing. It has been a humbling and rich experience to raise my children in a community that has reached out and supported women who have birthed. Birth blessings, food rosters for weeks after birthing when all the relatives have returned home, and the day-to-day care of your newborn and family kick off in earnest. Although it is not always easy to receive the gestures of loving generosity from friends and community, I encourage you to do so. It can be the first authentic experience of knowing that it truly does take a village to raise a child.

In Ayurveda, kichadi is the first food fed to a mother after she births in Ayurveda. This food has a nourishing, warming, and convalescing quality. After birthing, a woman's digestive warmth is diminished greatly. The body can be "cold" in this capacity and warmth is to be gently fueled to her, to rebuild the fire and rekindle her digestive flame. A space is created in the uterine cavity that can fill with air, regardless of whether the delivery was vaginal. This is to be pacified and taken care of for ongoing health in all aspects of a woman. Not only does it impact physically, but also emotionally and mentally. Plenty of ghee is given with the food to pacify, soothe, and nourish all the channels that have been opened, from the grossest to the subtlest, to facilitate the birth. Each and every cell has to land again and does so with a consciousness that was not possessed before the birth. You, as a woman, have changed. A threshold has been crossed and there is simply no return but a new path forward must be forged.

Fresh sprigs of dill are recommended to be eaten in the first few days after birthing. This herb facilitates efficient contraction of the uterus back to its natural size and quality of tissue. It does so gently and not forcefully. If the contracting tissue moves too fast, it will create discomfort.

I revere the cultures of our world that still honor the tradition of forty days rest for the mother after birthing. It saddens and concerns me beyond words when I see new mothers out and about within days of birthing. Yes, I understand some women feel isolated and lack family or community support to care for them and their children. However, people can reach out and ask for help. There is an army of women and men in your community just waiting to be called upon to help. Let them bring you some groceries, do school runs, hang the washing on the line. Your task is purely to convalesce and be fully immersed and absorbed with the miracle of life you have created. Please do not confuse your expanded state of love with physical energy to be out and engaged in worldly activity. Rest, dear woman. Rest. Again, each young woman, each daughter, is observing you and how you care for yourself. What are you teaching them?

Breastfeeding is sacred. You would not encourage your child or elderly relative to eat their meal while walking down a path. Why would women breastfeed an infant while walking down a path? I urge you to rest and feed in an environment conducive to your well-being and that of your infant.

Infertility

Conscious pregnancy is one of the most magical experiences of nature for a woman to have. To experience the power of creation within her own being as human life grows from the tissues of her own self, and often from a place of deep, instinctive feminine yearning. However, for many women since time began, and even more so for modern woman in contemporary living, pregnancy does not come effortlessly.

Infertility is a common health challenge for women and couples. And it's become big business, with health professionals specializing in this aspect of reproductive health.

There are so many contributing factors to infertility. Of them all, I consider stress to be number one. We are living in a world with overwhelming stress at this moment in time. Physiological, emotional, mental, environmental, collective planetary *stress*. My teacher in pulse reading used to say to patients, "You buy too much stress. You're buying from the wrong stall at the market. Here's your prescription, go to the next stall and buy a pound of ease and joy each week." It's true. We buy it, take it home, serve it up, and eat it! Stress adversely impacts a woman's reproductive health.

Fertility is the natural function of healthy hormonal processes and reproductive health. When the body is well and communication processes and flow are aligned, a woman generally experiences good fertility and endocrine health.

In Ayurveda it is considered infertility for a woman if problems exist that interfere with ovulation or block fallopian tube or implantation of the egg in the uterine wall; there has been consistent sex for twelve months without pregnancy; or there have been repeated miscarriages (known as habitual abortion).

Common physical causes of infertility can include:

- severe endometriosis
- pelvic inflammatory disease (PID)

- ovulation disorders
- elevated prolactin
- polycystic ovary syndrome (PCOS)
- early menopause
- benign uterine fibroids
- pelvic adhesions
- repeated miscarriages

CHAPTER 14

The Butterfly Years

. . . .

WHEN WE UNDERSTAND that there are governing forces in our body that are composed of the elements of nature, and rhythms that we dance to continuously throughout the day and night, then we come to understand a little more the simple ways that our body navigates its way through life. It's great to remember that we are so influenced by all we see, observe, and feel around us.

The phases of a woman's life change, for refined purpose and growth. Women have more drive in the pitta phase of life because of the motivation, drive, and will of this great generative force of energy. Although pitta may give more fire and ability to manifest, it can mean that, as women, we tend to push ourselves through obstacles and barriers, which can become a lifelong, deep-seated pattern without our even reflecting whether it truly supports us. It is easy to be habituated without consciously being aware of increasingly doing more and resting less. However, a woman's capacity to do, conquer, achieve, acquire, and accomplish naturally lessens as she ages and enters a vata-dominant phase of life.

When the body starts to change in perimenopause, it cannot maintain the pace of pushing and barging through obstacles. The drive of pitta reduces because of a change in its very nature as the dominant dośa. A woman can also have a hormonal imbalance and lack the nourishment to sustain the physical and mental capacity to meet life's challenges or even relate to them differently. If you push yourself too hard, it can be at the cost of going into deficit of your hormonal equilibrium, which affects the nourishment and health of all tissues in the body. If you are changing inwardly at one level and moving outwardly at another, discord will show up as disharmony. Women can experience this as suddenly questioning what they are doing with their life. We no longer have the physical drive to create, to manifest, and push. We become depleted and cracks appear, if we do try to keep pushing because we are not stable within ourselves. We don't have the inherent strength and capacity to just push on without rest and nourishment. Vata is wind and air, and it is erratic and irregular, so the aging phase is actually quite a catabolic stage of life, when tissue starts degenerating and breaking down.

The mental attributes of this stage of life are great intuitiveness, insightfulness, and all-knowingness. That's why these are the wisdom years. We become the great elder that nature intended. If we haven't looked after ourselves well, then it can be a very fearful, worrying, dark, heavy time. We weren't created by the divine to experience fear at this stage of life.

The reserve of reproductive hormones diminishes with menopause, such that you are less able to manage stress. It's like a physical reduction of your buffer zone, and this can show up more strongly in perimenopause if you are hormonally imbalanced. The greatest thing you can do is support yourself with nourishing practices. This support can be as simple as cultivating a daily meditation practice, inner reflection, and breathing exercises.

Ayurveda and yoga assist the sciences. Yoga is just so wonderful because it enhances all that we do. It fits so beautifully in the Ayurvedic paradigm because it creates space. Our body is all about communication that flows through spaces within us. If space is not created for that communication and flow to work efficiently, then we'll develop an imbalance, and symptoms will appear in the body.

Yoga creates physical, mental, emotional, and heart space for us to keep having clear perception, understanding, and good communication at every level of our being. This will translate as energy and stamina as well as enthusiasm for life.

It is all about balance, knowing when to push and when to pull back. These are the years of life for you to understand this, to live into "how" you ebb and flow with these rhythms.

You can barge along and push through life at the perimenopausal phase, but take great care unless you are well nourished, as the consequence of your actions will appear in the second half of your life, in menopause and beyond.

From the age of thirty-five, progesterone starts decreasing and reproductive hormones gradually diminish. Perimenopause can typically last between ten and fifteen years. In a healthy woman, it is asymptomatic. If you reduce and manage your stress, then you have enough nourishment in your hormones to be comfortable in menopause.

Flexibility is the golden key to wellness post-menopause. Observing nature and cycles, and surrendering to what the body needs, particularly in the menstrual years, is a good foundation for inward flexibility.

Why is physical and mental flexibility important? Well, it keeps you young at heart. Being able to adapt and respond to life as you meet it keeps your inner being soft and malleable. When you are rigid and inflexible, then contraction, fear, hardness, and degeneration come to you.

Ojas is the essence of your being and of vitality. It's the finest product of our tissues and our digestion. We go through the seven levels of tissue, the dhātus, and beyond the śukra dhātu is our ojas. The thing to understand about our ojas and tissues is that our tissues start at the grossest level. The deeper they go, the less they become in quantity and the more refined and qualitative. Hence, it is of great importance to nourish our tissues well, from the plasma right down to the reproductive tissue, and to keep our digestive processes functioning well so that our ojas, our vitality, is abundant and strong. When our ojas is depleted, our life force is weakened. When we do not have ojas, we do not have life.

In his book *Ayurveda for Women*, Dr. Robert Svoboda, an Ayurvedic physician says, "Menopause serves a woman's personal evolution for advancing. As we advance, ojas retreats. When it no longer contains sufficient ojas to contribute to production of new life, the woman's body shuts down reproductive capability and redirects its ojas to other projects."

What are the other projects? Well, beautiful woman, they are projects of a spiritual nature. The life forces that were so strongly established in uterine function now separate and become spiritualized forces. This is why balanced vata in this phase of life is about wisdom and insightfulness. Physically it is a sclerotic phase of degeneration, hardening, and aging. Our physical forces mineralize and harden, moving back toward the earth from which they are formed. This is nature, and how we are composed. Spiritually, it is a soulful part of your life. Therefore, dear ones, as you age, when you are in alignment, your spiritual forces move upward and back toward the cosmos from where they came. Depending on cultural circumstances, there may not be conscious awareness of these spiritual forces. They may not be revered, encouraged, or even fully understood to be put to meaningful use.

Fritz Helmut-Hemmerich in *Handbook of Anthroposophical Gynecology* describes the menopausal syndrome as follows. He says it is a dynamic in which bodily processes place decreasing demands on life forces. The continual activities of formation and transformation in the ovaries, fallopian tubes, cervix, and vagina, as well as in blood vessels and bones, are reduced or come to an end.

Thus the life forces become free for spiritual activities. In the context of social and cultural circumstances, however, these forces often cannot be put to meaningful use. During their change of life, women are expected to continue functioning more or less along customary lines.

We are seeing this more than ever in our culture. Also, because women have children later in life, they are still engaged strongly in the workforce and parenting while these processes of change are taking place, which can create absolute inner chaos and confusion.

Women are not given the reverence or support necessary, to nourish, step back, and become wise women, elders, and grandmothers in a gentle and sustainable way that nourishes and meets our needs to spiritualize.

Menopause

At menopause and beyond, vata is the mistress of imbalance. While vata moves and circulates all impulses and processes in the body, it also blocks and degenerates. Its nature is catabolic.

The mental and feeling qualities of vata, when harnessed, pacified and in harmony, are wisdom, intuitiveness, insight, truth.

The flip side, of course, when vata is aggravated, is fear, worry, anxiety, contraction, and narrowing. It is particularly important to pacify excess wind and gases, nourishing and calming the motion and quality of activity in the sensory and mental channels.

The commonly experienced difficulties and challenges for a woman at menopause are so prevalent and known to us in Western cultures that I really do not feel a need to share them. As a reminder, however, they include:

- heightened emotional sensitivity
- mental irritation, fear, anxiety, depression
- bloating and weight gain
- hot flashes, sweating, night sweats
- arthritis, stiffness, aches, pains
- osteopenia, osteoporosis

- disturbed sleep, unrefreshing sleep, insomnia
- dryness of the vaginal secretions and skin
- thinning hair
- sweating, night sweats
- prolapsed uterus
- memory loss, poor focus and concentration
- inability to hold stress, feeling of overwhelm

Even though hot flashes and night sweats or excessive sweating are heat related, they're due to vata imbalance at this junction, which sees you at a threshold. This junction takes solidity and steadfastness to know how to enter such crossing with wholeness and clarity. You are already whole and complete by your very nature, but you are called to remember the ways of living into it. This makes it a whole lot easier to enter this passage of menopause.

For so many women, however, vata imbalance means there is vulnerability as inner movement creates instability and cracks start to appear—sometimes small, vein-like cracks, and sometimes wide, deep chasms. The deeper and wider the crack, the more difficult to endure the transition.

The phase with hot flashes typically lasts twelve months. In 20 percent of women, though, this phase can last up to five long years. That's tough work and I know so many of you will be nodding in agreement here. This could have been your experience or the experience of women you know.

The greater the amount of pitta that has accumulated over the years, the more frequent, intense, and irritating will be the hot flashes, mood swings, and intense emotions. Now, this may sound somewhat disappointing and you may even sigh and slump, but there is no need, as you have the tools to establish harmony of your hormonal health. You can alleviate and even eliminate the potential of experiencing many or all of these symptoms. It is possible.

At the time of menopause, kapha can also be affected, which

means there can be weight gain, fluid retention, and swelling. This, too, is very common.

Judy, a fifty-two-year-old a musician, came to see me with hot flashes, night sweats, and tinnitus. Her sleep was disturbed, unrefreshing, and she was increasingly feeling performance anxiety before touring with a busy international schedule. She was lonely and wished for a life partner.

While Judy's metabolic heat was aggravated, we focused on pacifying her vata, bringing movement of it back down from its dominance in the nerve sensory system and mental channels, anchoring, grounding, and stabilizing her. Her treatment protocol included routine and rhythm, particularly around going to bed and rising. She followed the vata-pacifying diet and avoided sour and fermented foods. She began to do a daily self-oil massage. She was prescribed Ayurvedic herbal remedies. The remedies worked digestively on her physical, emotional, and mental bodies, breaking up blockages and pacifying aggravated vata, encouraging its correct path of movement. Herbs that work on breaking up blockages in circulatory channels grounded and nourished her emotional life, building her heart forces and supporting her biological rhythms. Herbs pacified her metabolic processes digestively and cooled the excess heat in the rakta dhātu, or blood.

Even though she expressed herself creatively through her music compositions and performances, Judy was encouraged to explore creative expression for fun. She took dance lessons, which brought her great joy and playfulness. In four months, her tinnitus reduced significantly, she no longer had night sweats, and her hot flashes were far less in frequency and intensity. She was able to compile, perform, and embrace new opportunities as a musician without anxiety and overwhelm. She created award-winning pieces of music, recorded, and found love in her life. Judy's light is shining like a bright star.

Remember you are the key to how you experience this change and you can make it better. How? Simply by following the lifestyle changes along with a pacifying diet as it applies to your constitution. You can do it, dear one. You and only you.

Balancing Vata

. . . .

Emphasizing breath and breath work pacifies and nourishes your vata. Prāṇāyāma and meditation are practices encouraged to support you in wellness. They keep the mental channels, nervous system, and impulses gentle and strengthened. Prāṇāyāma helps balance hormone and metabolic function.

When vata is balanced you may experience:

- enthusiasm
- good respiratory function
- alert body, mind, speech
- good transformation of tissues and movement of nutrients in the body
- creative imagination
- proper elimination of wastes, urine, stools, sweat
- balanced nervous system

Signs and symptoms of imbalanced vata are:

- confusion, emptiness of head, memory loss
- bladder incontinence, constipation, chronic fatigue or tiredness
- less oxygen to the body because of respiratory blockages
- aches, pains, muscular body stiffness and joint problems
- fear, anxiety, depression
- loss of appetite, vitality, stamina
- hypothyroidism or low secretions of any organ
- very talkative but unable to listen
- tremors
- dryness of the skin, hair and mouth
- phobias of all kinds, including of the dark, heights, social situations
- light sleep, restless sleep
- degenerative diseases like osteopenia, osteoporosis, arthritis

To reduce vata, follow a vata-reducing diet (see the guidelines in appendix B). Avoid eating too much raw food, dried fruit, gas-producing foods (fermented, dry, crunchy), white sugar, heavy beans (kidney beans, lima beans, and chickpeas), dry crackers, corn chips, potatoes, and cabbage.

Eat more: sweet fruits and melons; cooked vegetables, especially pumpkin, zucchini, and squashes; ghee; buttermilk; honey; jaggery; coconut sugar; white meat; red lentils; yellow mung, adzuki beans and whole green mung; olive oil; coconut oil.

Here are some home remedies for excess vata.

For stiffness and aching joints: Take one teaspoon of castor oil and sip hot ginger tea before bed. Castor oil pacifies vata, so it calms the degenerative forces.

For swelling and pain: Mix and take with a half teaspoon of warm water daily:

1 tsp ground turmeric

¼ tsp garlic juice

¼ tsp ground ajwain

½ tsp ground coriander

½ tsp ground fenugreek

The R's

The Sanskrit sound for the letter R is an inward sound. Here, I wish to remind you of the R's: rest, repose, reflect, remember, revere, renew, recalibrate, reverberate, resonate. These are daily activities of nourishment to have in your life.

The world needs you to recognize your intrinsic requirement for this deep nourishment. To step up, step in, and own your womanhood. To allow yourself to naturally evolve into this phase of wisdom. To allow yourself to be the elder, the storyteller. It's the sum of all your life experiences and stories up until this point that is necessary as a meaningful contribution to life. There is a natural order of things, and when you step up, you nourish our daughters, our granddaughters, and show them the way of being, teach them the essence of the Great Feminine. She is not hard and pounding. She is soft, gentle, and light. If you constantly flap too hard, you'll be like a one-sided bird with a really heavy and sore wing, flapping around in circles. There needs to be a balance here.

It is for all mothers, all daughters, and Mother Earth that we do this for ourselves. We have a sacred duty to ourselves to be nourished.

Stella, a fifty-six-year-old teacher, came to see me. She was tired of being tired! She was overweight and could not shed the excess pounds. Life was good, but she felt there was a certain kind of spark lacking. She felt a great sense of selfishness. Even in seeing me, she felt selfish. Even as a child she was told she was selfish. She had a lot of fluid retention in the tissues, and sluggish metabolic processes and digestion.

We used herbs and diet to bolster these, and reduce the swelling and retention of fluid, creating an inner spaciousness for her to feel more life energy. She cleansed one day a week with mung soup. I gave her an aurum rose lavender cream to apply to her heart region, which worked on building the subtle heart forces and gave a sense of gentle, loving nourishment. In her belief that she was selfish, she was not living in reciprocal relationship: She was giving but not receiving. After three months she had more energy and spark. Her body did not feel heavy, her metabolism was slowly recalibrating. The greatest internal shift was in how she consciously created strategies to meet her needs to be nourished without feeling selfish. She took accrued paid leave for a school term and focused on doing what gave her a sense of deep nourishment and purpose.

Understanding this composition of nourishment and what it means is an important task for you as a woman. I encourage you to complete Enrichment Activity #7 in appendix F to contemplate the kind of nourishment you feed yourself daily. Consider its essence. What does it mean to you? What are you really feeding yourself? What purpose is your nourishment serving in your life?

CHAPTER 15

Connectedness and Flow

· · · · · · · · · · · · ·

IN THE BEGINNING is love, in the end is love, and in the middle, we have to cultivate love. I believe that women are seeking deep connectedness in their yearning for self-love.

There are ways of cultivating virtues that create, sustain, and maintain an inner flow, keeping you connected to self. This is a refined and qualitative place to reach in terms of your life processes. It really is about tending your inner garden, your connection to self and unimpeded flow. You need to cultivate this space so that you can flourish. We can observe this flourishing externally in nature, mirrored in your own inner nature.

A wonderful tool with which to cultivate and maintain this connection is the "Triple C" framework for connectedness to yourself: clarity, compassion, and communication. You can visualize this framework as a triangle with the virtues of clarity, compassion, and communication at each point. Your pulsating essence and vitality exist within the triangle. This innermost space represents being, your connection.

You can choose to cultivate the quality of your mental channels, anchoring you in radiance and vitality. No matter what is going on in your life, even when in the eye of a big shitstorm!

Ultimately the greatest virtue you are cultivating is love.

Listen, great woman. Listen to the inner hum.
The sound that resonates as you cultivate connectedness and flow.
The sound of your inner sanctum, your innermost garden.
The connectedness to your womanhood.
To the great indwelling teacher, I offer gratitude.
She is the one who understands you and knows all.
The one who knows you so intimately and your innermost nature.

The Triple C Framework

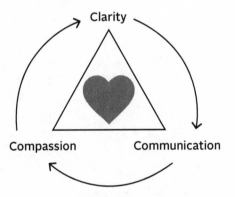

When there is a structure or framework, it creates a scaffolding within ourselves in which we are able to grow, sustain, blossom, and thrive.

The Triple C is a scaffolding for your inner qualities of clarity, compassion, and communication to be able to cultivate and grow throughout your life, particularly through phases of life that see challenge, transition, and change. These phases may be depleting, fatiguing, stressful and may dry out your vital juices.

The three C's are based on qualities that cultivate self-love. When you have an abundance of self-love, you can have more peacefulness and ease, greater love for others, and greater love for life.

It starts with listening to yourself. When you are able to observe yourself, observe what you are feeling, giving your attention and focus to such feelings, being able to recognize and articulate these feelings, then you can start to look at your underlying needs. The needs behind your feelings are not only unique to you or me but also are universal human needs that we all share.

When you can recognize and become familiar with your basic needs, then you can adjust and change to have these needs met. These are small, simple steps for change but, over time, powerful change that establishes you in yourself. You can become more established in your own empowered true nature, giving you laser-sharp, penetrating, unwavering *clarity*. Where there is clarity, your decision making is easier. The cloud of confusion lifts.

When I am confused, invariably it is because I simply do not have enough or the right information. Where there is connectedness and flow, the very movement gives crystal clarity from moment to moment because such movement possesses the right rhythm. Having the right information about what you feel and need creates the alignment for clarity. Then you can choose to take the right action that nourishes and cultivates this very love at the core of your essence.

Otherwise, life can become exhausting. It is so loud and stressful in the world. Sometimes, it's so loud that you cannot even feel clear on what you need to wear, eat, or read, on which way to turn at a crossroads, on what kind of exercise to take, on how to relate to yourself and others... the list goes on and on, with infinite possibilities. It can feel endless.

Confusion sucks up a lot of fuel. It takes so much energy to be confused. It's exhausting! Clarity, though, gives energy. When you are clear, you feel more balanced, more aligned, harmonious and open. You feel more present. Not in the past, not in the future, but present in this moment. In this way, you can have *compassion* for yourself. This is a nourishment of yourself with empathy flowing in. This is listening to yourself. You must be gentle to do such listening.

It takes great strength to be gentle, and as women we know strength. Each of you is strong beyond compare. The power of strength in you is utterly formidable. However, strength can be harsh, abrasive, abrupt, even forceful. This is not the kind of strength I am writing of. I am referring to the great virtue of gentleness, which feeds your self-compassion. And it is only when you have an abundance of compassion for yourself that you are able to have empathy for others.

The golden rule of compassionate communication, of Marshall Rosenberg's Nonviolent Communication (NVC), is that you cannot give empathy when you are most in need of it yourself. How can you have a broad bandwidth without this? It is not possible, not sustainable, and is absolutely lacking in nourishment. This is not passive and abundant in a way you can receive. You cannot offer your cup to quench the thirst of another when it is empty, just as you first take sustenance from the chalice before sharing it with another.

When you have clarity and compassion, you can experience authentic, loving, effective, and conscious *communication*. Again, the body is a series of channels all about communication, process and flow.

Communication (from the Latin *commūnicāre*, meaning "to share") is the act of conveying intended meaning from one entity or group to another through the use of mutually understood signs. The main step inherent to all communication is forming a communicative motivation or reason. There is an intention behind all communication.

The motivation behind communication is love and being alive. Communication has the potent possibility of being a healing gesture or harming gesture.

As a woman, this is all about how things share, move, form, and love within you and from you. It's all about how you perceive, experience, share, serve, and love in the world.

These three C's connect you with yourself, your self-love, and your feminine essence. A woman connected with self-love and feminine essence in all phases of her womanhood is an Ayurvedic woman. You can wear these three C's like a sacred feminine armor, shielding you for life!

Mantras and Healing

Your nervous system and nerve sense activity are supported and cultivated by the qualities of connectedness, flow, and ease. In essence, your nervous system has two parts:

- the sympathetic nervous system: your fight-flight-freeze, or stress response
- the parasympathetic nervous system: your repair-rest-digest response

The sympathetic nervous system is crucial for survival of the human being. It's what kicked in instinctively and kept our ancestors safe and alive. Without it, we would not be here! It is clever in keeping us safe.

In sympathetic mode, energy gets pulled fast into your core. It pulls and grips, tightening the organs to the front of the spine and creating a state of hypervigilance. This is why you can feel it strongly in your very gut when in fight-or-flight mode. It has the capacity to increase your heart rate and breathing, and mobilize your arms and legs so that you can run away or fight. It causes the eyes to scan rapidly, broadening your scope of vision. Thus, it is difficult to focus cognitively and be present when in fight-flight-freeze mode.

Today we have a chronic challenge of discerning between daily pressures of life and mortal danger. Our sympathetic nervous system is activated too frequently for many people, by any form of constantly perceived stress. It does not matter whether it's a bill in the mail, not being invited to morning tea or a social activity, having no likes on social media, or discovering a venomous snake underfoot and ready to strike. These can all be perceived as stressors. For women, there are so many stressors. One could be not being physically present to help a child, neighbor, or friend in need. It may be not having food to feed your family or not knowing that there will always be a roof over your head and that you will be provided for.

But because these daily stressors, these triggers, are constant and prevalent for most of us, we're chronically unable to enter a state of physiological rest. This consumes vitality. The health and integrity of your tissues and organs are consumed, too, when the opportunity to renew lacks in quality and quantity.

Our parasympathetic nervous system is responsible for our innate healing. The healing mechanisms belong to this realm of rest-repair-digest. For example, when you are ill, if you get good quality rest, you recover much faster and with greater integrity.

Vitality and vibrancy come from the restorative processes of the parasympathetic nervous system: mentally, emotionally, and physically. Feeling safe in your skin, feeling safe in your life and in the world are essential for the parasympathetic nervous system to function.

Sanskrit mantras are a most effective tool for cultivating a sense of safety, fullness, and inner freedom. Mantra practice works on the quality of your mind. The resonance of the sounds of mantras stimulates the parasympathetic nervous system. Sanskrit is the language of vibration and resonance. Please see appendix G, Notes on the Transliteration and Pronunciation of Sanskrit, for more details and guidance. The way the sounds are pronounced sends a resonance throughout your entire being, for sound has particular meaning and quality.

You can heal from trauma and overwhelm and become creatively enlivened. When you get a better grip on the control button, you can switch between the sympathetic fight-or-flight and parasympathetic rest-repair function. The stronger your muscle is built to flick the switch on and off, the better you can heal from trauma, stressors, and living in perpetual overwhelm.

Here are some tools for care of the parasympathetic nervous system to support this:

- Meditate regularly: Establishing yourself in the regular practice of meditation builds the muscle of being able to rest-repair and replenish. Then it becomes a more familiar way of being and helps you navigate life responsively, not constantly reactively, as you do in fight-flight-freeze. (Ways of meditating include mantra *japa*, yoga *nidra*, restorative yoga, yin yoga, tai chi, and chi gong).

- Get good quality sleep.

- Stay hydrated and regularly cleanse to release accumulated toxins and inflammation created by the stress hormones adrenaline and cortisol. Drinking fresh veggie juices is a great way to support this, as it keeps the plasma and lymph well hydrated and clean.

- Drink ghee mixed in hot water in the morning.

- Give yourself a self-oil massage, or *abhyanga*. When you massage with warm oil before bathing it is pacifying for the nervous system.

- Take foot baths with lavender oil and/or Epsom salts.

- Do prāṇāyāma (breathing exercises).

- Engage in art therapy.

Growth and Maturation

> The one within the body, when she has
> discovered the true nature of the self, shines.
> Shines radiant bliss.
> **UPANISHADS**

As you grow and mature as a woman, you are called to live from your heart's intelligence, creating the story of your life and telling the story you dream of living. Maturation is about blossoming and allowing your radiance to blossom. This kind of growth is about being connected to the sound of your womanhood, the pulsating sound that throbs in your very being and knows the entirety of the unknown.

Guide me to the purpose for which I am born on the Earth.
My balance is secure in the hands of God.
Help my life to fulfill this purpose. Grant me to have all power
and wisdom that I may best fulfill my life's purpose.
O spirit of guidance. Throw thy divine light on my path.
Open my heart that thy spirit it may reflect. My mind is still.
My thought is steady. My sight is keen.
Make thy heart thy divine temple.
HAZRAT INAYAT KHAN

How do you activate your wisdom to remain fully vital? How do you blossom as you live from this place of heart wisdom and emotional intelligence once it has been created?

Just as the Native American proverb says:

Listen to the wind, it speaks.
Listen to the silence, it speaks.
Listen to your heart, it knows.

In essence, dear woman, this is it. This is what it's all about. All you seek and yearn for lies in listening to your heart. Your heart knows. It knows what you need, your yearning, your greatness, your purpose. Your heart knows your pain, your lack, your burdens. Your heart knows that you are a unique creation of the divine who needs you, to express purposefully through you, in a way that only you can.

This is why Ayurveda was gifted to humanity, so that we can establish ourselves in our listening. To remember how to listen, to listen to the complete wisdom of the universe that is contained within us because we are it. There is in fact no difference between you and universal energy. It is all energy in different forms. How it moves, works, feels, experiences is a dance. It's all a dance of creation. It's full on. But this is what it is, and the substance it is composed of is the substance of love.

You are whole and complete in essence. Life is a play of consciousness: mysterious, bizarre, and the play of creation and life.

Tantric philosophy offers a means to grasp this concept of the play of life. Tantra is a kind of science, a way of knowledge for understanding the outer world and the inner world of the human psyche. It is associated with Ayurveda and Vedic astrology, along with alchemical traditions through the medieval worlds of China, India, the Middle East, and Europe. In fact, it's the basis of much European mysticism.

Tantra encompasses the creation of the universe, destruction of the universe, worship of the divine, attainment of goals in life and spiritual powers. It embodies ways of meditation to realize your ultimate truth—the truth of who you are as a woman, the truth of womankind.

O Goddess, Lord Śiva, having created the sixty-four tantras
to confuse the entire world to become dependent upon
external powers, again by your word brought down your tantra,
which gives self-reliance and fulfils at once all the aims of life.
SHANKARACHARYA, SAUNDARYA LAHARI

The quality of a woman's life force can be looked at like the dhā-tus, the seven tissues in the body. The grossest tissue, rasa, which is plasma and lymph, has the most quantity. The finest tissue, śukra, the reproductive tissue, is far less in quantity, but is more refined in its quality and essence. This, too, is occurring in you as a woman as you mature and grow.

When you give attention to feeding your inner life and cultivating your inner garden, you are able to experience the deepest inner beauty. This is authentic beauty, not beauty that is mistaken, Rājasic, or outwardly driven, and unstable, ultimately creating disharmony. This is sāttvic beauty. It is inward, harmonious and balanced.

This time of life has a particular quality of illumination that is your radiance and vitality. When you live into this, you are a radiant woman. You are the essence of the Ayurvedic woman. You are consciously aware of the substance and gesture of woman. It is absolute, for you have remembered your nature and established yourself in your radiance.

Ultimately this is what the second half of life is about: becoming your wisdom. It is about doing less and being more. It's about becoming more refined, expending your energy more wisely and in measured, refined ways.

CHAPTER 16

The Wise Woman Years

· · · · · · · · · · · · ·

THE YEARS OF a woman's life beyond the transformation she undergoes in menopause see a divine establishment in her maturation of self. As the vata phase of life becomes dominant, the aging forces prevail. A woman is anchored by the mineral forces of her body and illumined by the light of spiritual orientation so active by nature. This is woman's natural deep inner beauty radiating in full effulgence. What a joy it is to inhale the company of one who takes their place in such a regal manner. The physical body may shrink and wither, dry out, lose strength and malleability, but the light from within grows stronger and brighter. This is, of course, when a woman allows such light to organically, without resistance, illumine her emergence as the elder.

When I was seven years of age I knew I wanted
to grow up to become a wise woman.
A MENTOR

Do What Lights You Up

Your second half of life is lived as a storyteller. You've dropped your stories to become your wisdom and this is the greatest story ever to be told. This is the story the world needs, the story of your life's purpose. This is the story the world is waiting for, the story to be shared with children. It's the story that daughters, girls, young women, women of all ages, stages, and phases need to hear, to be nourished and guided by. Your story is important.

Only you can tell it because it is unique to you. It was gifted to you by the divine. It has a quality that can only come in the right season. A tree or plant will not blossom out of season. It goes against the very nature of the tree to do so. And so it is with you.

Listening is needed to become this wisdom. It commands you to listen to the heart and that means making spaciousness in your life. If the second half of life sees you live at a pace that is frantic for you, working super-hard and feeling that you are not getting anywhere, or pulling you in many directions, then your listening cannot be fully known. If there are many expectations of you to meet rent, crunch numbers in your job, make the sales, market, promote, do tasks and work that feels mundane and holds no spiritual meaning, beauty, or value for you, then it's so much harder to cultivate the virtues of self-care, compassion, communication, and self-love. It is harder to cultivate the necessary inner spaciousness you require.

Unfold your own myth.
JALĀL AL-DĪN MUHAMMAD RŪMĪ

You can still contribute, accomplish, manifest, run a business, and work effectively. But you are called to work more wisely, with greater refinement and understanding.

This phase is all about quality. The capacity for quantity is not so prevalent by its very nature. Hence, there's an inability to multitask, juggle, and hold so many things at once as effortlessly as you once could. For there's a prevalent inner drive and yearning to simplify, to get connected with the greater quality of all you are and do. It's about your relationships. First and foremost, it's about your relationship to yourself, dear woman.

What feeds your vitality, harmony, and ease here is creative expression. It is how you can offer and give expression to who you are.

There are endless possibilities to express yourself creatively. This is because every action you take can be a creative expression when it is connected with your heart. Each breath can be a creative expression. It's key that your creative expression is nourished and fed by action that has meaning for you—something that lights you up and sparks a flame inside of you, something that makes you feel alive and activates you.

Finding activities that light you up is creative expression. This is what you do with your blossoming. You may simply express each gesture infused with connection to your heart, with love. If only it were that simple to establish yourself in this place!

Yet, dear one, your creative expression is the very gesture of your citti, your consciousness. And this is the only thing you take with you when you leave your physical body. That's good motivation to do all that you can to live as a creative expression of the divine. And to ensure the quality of your citti is not too shitty!

It's simple. Do what truly lights you up.

A dear friend and colleague many years ago shared with me that she had an opportunity to dance in her son's school performance. Being a dutiful mother, she reluctantly consented, only to experience a whole new vista open within herself. There was joy and passion through the expression of the dance. She realized that she had been working so hard in building a successful business, for decades, but without doing anything creative purely for fun. She began to dance and dance, feeling joy and fulfilment in a way that had been lacking within her heart for years.

Similarly, when my youngest daughter was a babe in arms, I was at a local fair watching a community African drum and dance group perform. I could see the passion and inner beauty in each person in the group. They were truly having fun and I thought, *that's for me*. I ultimately did join that group and sang, drummed, did percussion, dressed up in traditional African clothing, and danced. It was so much fun and lit me up in a way that enlivened my entire being. I was not the greatest drummer, or the most fluent and coordinated dancer, definitely not the most flowing or articulate group member, but I was tapping into a life force within me that was so vital. I just loved the dance. I was expressing myself creatively and palpably grounding myself, bringing myself out of my thoughts, into my heart, and simultaneously into metabolic bliss. Tapping into life force. My hormones were very happy.

Journaling is a great thing to do because writing is a cathartic process and we express our heart through our hand and word. It's a creative expression beyond words. You do not have to be a wordsmith. It's pure creative consciousness coming through your hand into words on a page. That's it! It's beautiful and sacred.

For this reason, I always encourage journaling. I've worked with women who do not feel safe to write for fear it will be read. If that applies to you then write it and destroy it. The creative expression comes in the very *act* of writing. The product does not have to be kept. Your dreams cannot come to fruition if they are never put on the page. It's just not possible unless they are written.

It's really about discerning what is alive in your heart, knowing what your heart is longing for. Knowing what lights you up, being in touch with what ignites your passion and keeps you feeling enlivened. Universally, all our needs are fundamentally similar. Their expression, how they manifest, looks unique to each of us. This is our creative expression. It is born from the heart.

In a woman, the seat of creative expression is in uterine health. This is an outward expression of your sound, of your cosmic signature, the song of your own symphony and of your womanhood. It gives you pure imagination and feeds your capacity to dream. This is why it is to be fostered and revered. It is pure. It is truth. And it will only, can only, speak to you when you listen to it.

In the second half of life, if you cannot, will not, are not listening, then menopause can be rough and problematic. All kinds of health challenges that deplete you of your radiance and vitality can prevail and plague you.

So you must try not to block your potential, your spaciousness, flow, and connection to an infinite field of possibility for your life.

This point of growth is deep and refined. When likened again to the seven levels of tissue of the body, this is the majja dhātu: the cells of the bone marrow. Osteogenesis of cells happens here and how you feed bone marrow is really significant, as it is key to rejuvenation. Ayurveda says that the effect of good bone marrow on the tissues of the mind and emotions is a sweet resonance that is respected by all. It is soft and composed.

Foods that nourish bone marrow (so you could say, foods that support growth and maturation in you) are walnuts, dried fruits (soaked is better, to rehydrate and make them easier on digestion), almonds, pistachios, coconut, ghee, pumpkin and squash, zucchini, pomegranate, cumin, sesame seed, soy milk (if tolerated and good quality non-GMO), unhomogenized cow milk.

To know what your heart is calling for, to allow the dreaming of the heart to come forth, you peel off the layers. You remove the veils that separate you from yourself intimately and clearly, the very layers that have accumulated over a lifetime of hurts, pains, rejections, not being enough, not looking inward and putting attention outward, not listening, not feeling accepted or loved.

Before you speak, it is necessary for you to listen,
for God speaks in the silence of the heart.
MOTHER TERESA

Here are the tools of Ayurveda that support listening to your
heart's calling effectively:

- Diet (to pacify according to your constitution)

- *Panchakarma* therapies (massage therapies, heart *dharas* and heart
  pichus) (These are therapeutic treatments in which warm medicated oils and decoctions are poured and, in the latter, soaked over
  the center of the chest, the region of your feeling heart.)

- Herbs (Those that work on the feeling heart and remove the
  blocks. Herbs that penetrate and break up the layers and peel
  back the veils, nourish and build up heart forces, nourish and pacify the feeling heart, bring clarity, bring the impulse for creative
  expression and life force, connectedness to self and self-love.)

- Creams (Rub creams that build the heart forces into your heart,
  give protective sheaths and shield yourself. Allow to let die what
  no longer serves and birth regularly the new.)

- Yoga āsana (to maintain the inner spaciousness and inner flexibility to yoke)

- Mantra (Use sacred sound syllables that work on the quality of
  mind. "Hallelujah," "amen," "auṁ namaḥ Śivāya" "so'ham" all
  work—whatever is sacred to you!)

- Breath (prāṇāyāma)

- Meditation

- Prayer

In following your life's purpose comes the clarity to feel more courageous and pursue what your soul is drawn to do. There is greater capacity to create and manifest, to give expression, to allow yourself to be, to take ownership of yourself, to be enough, to love, to be loved, to accept, to embody, to embrace, to celebrate.

My teacher's guru, Baba Ramdas Swami, used to say that there are three things to achieve in life:

- One: Know what you want.
- Two: Achieve what you want.
- Three: Enjoy what you have achieved.

He would say:

- 95 percent of people on the planet do not know what they want.
- 3 percent of people know what they want but they cannot achieve it.
- 1 percent of people know what they want, achieve what they want, but cannot enjoy it.
- 1 percent of people know what they want, achieve what they want, and enjoy what they achieve.

Most of us do not even know what we really want. It is difficult to be so clear that you know, be so clear that you can manifest in action, be so connected that you can enjoy what you've achieved.

Using these tools and doing these practices gives greater opportunity to be one of the 1 percent. Remember that Ayurveda gifted these tools to humanity. Receive and use the gifts well!

Marma Chikitsa

Marma is a powerful instrument. It works on energy junctions in the body: the physical, the mental, the emotional, the conscious, the subconscious. It creates focus, awareness, alertness, healing, firmness, and emotional and mental flexibility. It lets you be flexible about your beliefs and values, to expand and adapt as you grow. Marma allows you to go beyond your comfort zone.

Marma clears the canvas. It puts perceptions, interpretations, your "what happened," and your stories back where they belong—in the filing cabinet. It allows the reinvention of your true success.

When you work with marma points for the mind, you create an opportunity for clear perception, which lets you make new possibilities regularly.

Certain kinds of toxins can block mental channels. Marma removes the blocks, and toxins are released from these mental channels. Then, the *buddhi* (which is the conscious and subconscious mind) is stimulated. You can communicate directly with your buddhi. Marma helps to create effective communication.

MARMA FOR FOCUS, CONCENTRATION, AWARENESS, AND ENERGY

Use your left hand at the back of your head to cradle your occiput. Place your right index finger just above your top lip in the little groove. Gently but with focused intention, press this point six times. You can repeat this, but always press the point in patterns of six and always use the same finger. Press this point for instant alertness. When you press this point, oxygen goes to the brain. You are clearing and oxygenating mental channels.

EKĀGRACITTA MARMA

Ekāgracitta is one-pointed focus. Doing ekāgracitta daily strengthens your feeling heart. It makes you emotionally stronger and fortifies your emotional intelligence. It builds your one-pointed focus and presence so that you are able to see, listen, perceive more clearly. It lets you to respond more fully from a place of total presence. Even in the midst of chaos, you can remain steadfast in your presence.

Ekāgracitta can be done by making a black, circular dot the size of a small coin (just under an inch in diameter) in the center of a small card, such as a blank recipe card.

Take a firm posture. If you are sitting in a chair, place both feet evenly in power position on the floor. If you are sitting on the ground or floor, please be mindful that you are upright with a strong, elongated spine.

Using both hands, hold the card up in front of your face and slowly move it away from your face, in front of you, focusing on the dot in the center of the card.

The object of this exercise is to look at the dot for three minutes without blinking. If you blink, start again. Initially, you may only be able go without blinking for thirty seconds or less. Your eyes may burn, ache, and become uncomfortable. It's okay. You are building a muscle here. Persist.

Over time, you will be able to focus on the dot for longer periods, up to three minutes (more if you wish).

When you finish, place down the card and close your eyes for a few minutes.

If preferred, you may also do this exercise using a candle flame. I find the dot most effective, portable, and it can be used anywhere.

You will find that, over time, whatever is going on around you, you are able to stay focused on the dot (or flame) without being distracted. You will be aware of what is happening, but your attention will stay fixed.

THE "FORGIVE-AND-FORGET" MARMA POINT

The right brain can work well only when left (the past) is complete. When you are not complete with your past, when unable to digest past experiences, which accumulate as a sludge-like substance on the receptors of the brain and mental channels and in the channels of the feeling heart, then new life is blocked. The past moves forward into the present by way of accumulation. This forgive-and-forget marma point allows you to file the past where it needs to be and to let new life potential enter you.

On your left hand at the web between the thumb and index finger is a natural indentation that is a marma point. Pressing this point six times, in intervals, up to a few minutes. Sitting quietly with eyes closed, observe what and who comes up, and let it go. Let go of the hurts that burden you and prevent your full maturation.

These are ancient, penetrating, powerful tools that allow you to work with your inner spaciousness, maturation, and wisdom. You keep working on and expanding your awareness qualitatively. These marma points help to do this.

Every part of you has a secret language.
Your hands and your feet say what you have done.
And every need brings in what's needed.
Pain bears its cure like a child.
Having nothing produces provisions.
Ask a difficult question,
And the marvelous answer appears.
JALĀL AL-DĪN MUHAMMAD RŪMĪ

CHAPTER 17

Your Legacy

. . . .

WHAT IS YOUR offering and contribution to life? What harvest are you bringing to the table of life? What is your legacy and how do you spread the seeds of your service? Contribution and selfless service have such virtue, as they are a pure expression of self-love, offering without expectation or attachment, your love in action.

In this very moment you may acknowledge yourself. You are *pūrṇam*, perfect. You are whole and complete in essence. Nothing can make you less whole and complete than you already are. This is your unchanging state, your womanhood.

I invite you to consciously invoke your wisdom, your indwelling teacher, to show you your gifts, your seeds of service, the seeds you spread and sow. This is your legacy.

Use the tools and practices in this book to become present to your authenticity. This all-knowingness is your healer and healing, your most holistic physician, your deep inner beauty, your gift, the sound of your radiance. Dear one, now is the moment to really listen to your womanhood.

Allow these words to move through you:

The roar of joy that set the world in motion
Is reverberating in your body
And the space between all bodies.
Beloved, listen.
Find that exuberant vibration
Rising new in every moment,
Humming in your secret places,
Resounding through the channels of delight.
Know you are flooded by it always.
Float with the sound.
Melt with it into divine silence.
The sacred power of space will carry you
Into the dancing radiant emptiness
That is the source of all.
The ocean of sound is inviting you
Into its spacious embrace,
Calling you home.
Immerse yourself in the rapture of music.
You know what you love. Go there.
Tend to each note, each chord,
Rising up from silence and dissolving again.
Vibrating strings draw us
Into the spacious resonance of the heart.
The body becomes light as the sky
And you, one with the Great Musician,
Who is even now singing us
Into existence.

YUKTI VERSES 16 AND 18, *THE RADIANCE SUTRAS*

Your legacy is really about contemplating what you offer in your life. It is about the gifts you possess and how you share these with others. As you mature and grow, as you age and embody your wisdom, as you establish yourself as an elder, you share these gifts.

These gifts are insight, knowledge, truth; how to cultivate virtues; how to be a good, kind person; how to love; how to respect; how to see beauty; how to know yourself; how to care for nature; how to create, sustain, maintain, sow, grow, and harvest; how to rest; how to let go; how to surrender that which keeps you limited.

What resonates in these gifts you share, of this legacy, of this offering, is the sound of your offering. It has a musical quality, like a song that you love to listen to. Throughout life, this song takes you to a place of remembrance, longing, inspiration, joy, fun, love—growth, but a song.

So I ask you to think about the sound of your legacy. What is the sound of your contribution? As a woman, what is your legacy to daughters, to granddaughters, to young women, mothers, aunties, sisters, to all women?

Long before the soul incarnates, it is sound.
It is for this reason that we love sound.
HAZRAT INAYAT KHAN

There must be purpose to your incarnating. There must be a song, a story. Like any great fable or tale, there is meaning. The essence of the story teaches us. It shows us the way. It allows us to contemplate and resonate with a place of knowing in us. It stirs something into wakefulness.

In *The Radiance Sutras*, Lorin Roche says, "Immerse yourself in the rapture of music. You know what you love. Go there." What is the "there"? What does it look like to you? What is it that lights you up, that has always lit you up? What is it that keeps your flame burning brightly, that has fueled your longing in life and satisfied your insatiable hunger? What makes deep sense and is truth to you? What gives meaning to you?

When you are nourishing that very place in you, that "there," then you are in flow, you are connected. When you are connected, you cannot help but be of contribution and service. This is your very nature, the absolute nature of woman. The "create and give," the reciprocal relationship.

And in the processes of life and nature, this spirit of service truly comes into its own in the most mature phase of life.

If we look at a plant, it begins as a seed with unlimited potential for growth. This seed must first be planted. In nature, the very plant from which the seed was born is what has released it and allowed the elements of nature to spread and grow it. Moved by the wind, sewn into the earth, moistened by water, warmed by the sun, all enabled by the existence of space—these are the very elements we live by.

The seed requires the right conditions to grow. It requires the right season, cycle, rhythms conducive for its unique growth.

The seed begins to grow. At first, it's a tiny shoot. It grows strong. Upward toward the light, deep into the ground, rooted by its very nature and fed by the minerals of the earth. It takes in light. It takes in warmth. It takes in moisture. It eliminates what it does not need and what does not serve it. It takes in nourishment. It does not hold back in its growth. It is connected and flows. It matures and blossoms. It bears its fruit. It peaks. Then, like its very nature, the plant releases its seeds. The seeds that contain its very essence may live on and regenerate. These are its gifts and contribution, its legacy.

And so it is with you. Whether you are conscious of this or not, you are creating a legacy. You are contributing the fruits of your harvest and this is what you bring to the table to share with others.

This is not something to be measured by quantity, but just like the tissues, or dhātus, of the body, your legacy is to be valued by its most refined essence, its quality. The most refined quality or essence in you is your ojas. In this way, your vitality can be linked with your contribution. This is the very song of your womanhood. It's a story unique to you. It is meant for you. It is the story of your life and your experience and perception of life. It emanates from you.

Sharing your stories is a contribution and impactful. Your stories, when shared, teach others that they may grow and learn. Your stories are alive. Your stories mentor others. When you connect, collaborate with your family, your circle, your community, you are contributing simply by sharing your stories.

**She who knows the secret of the sound, knows
the mystery of the whole universe.**
HAZRAT INAYAT KHAN

This is a reciprocal part of nature. Just as you have grown and been fed the right sustenance by stories of others, you, too, are called to share yours. They are needed and necessary in all phases, from early childhood right through life. When a child is in the mother's womb, the mother will tell stories to the child. When somebody dies, at the funeral service and wake stories of the person's life are shared. There is an innate quality in the sharing of these stories. The magic that happens here, the alchemical processes occur through the live transmission of your essence, your sound, when you share. The resonance of this music is received by those you share with. This resonance is all that remains after you are gone.

The phases of life support these processes. The kapha phase is the planting of a seed and then relying on the earth and water elements. Pitta is the activating, creating, manifesting through warmth and fire. The vata phase is the maturation and wisdom of experience, releasing the seeds and enabling them to spread.

These are, just like Ayurveda teaches us, the principles of nature and how they play out in each season of life. They allow us to experience our task and the nature of our feminine self.

When you live in alignment with your nature, when you are using the right tools for creating and maintaining your vitality, then by nature you are contributing, you are spreading the seeds of your inherent gifts, for it is your nature to do so. This just happens naturally when you are connected to yourself. It is not forced or hard, but simply happens.

You do not have to force. You do not have to become anything you are not already. You simply have to reveal your inner treasure, your light. Your light is the essence of your contribution. Your light is what you bring to the table and what you leave as a legacy.

Let's consider ways to support this light.

The Gratitude Journal

Keep a gratitude journal. Regularly write a list of all the things that you are grateful for in your day. Reflect on the great blessings and grace you have in your life, seeing what you have, all you are, and celebrate yourself with the love generated by gratitude. Gratitude generates so much love, self-worth and esteem. It feeds your vitality. When you have such gratitude, you are open and flowing. You simply generate kindness and love in its very sharing. Your light kindles the light in others.

Reflection

Contemplate your values.

Reflect on the values that are alive in you now. They regularly change. The values that hold significance and meaning for you might be: love, family, faith, acceptance, community, creativity, responsibility, discovery, vision, collaboration, gratitude, perception, consciousness, completion, organization, efficiency, cleanliness, spiritual hygiene, order, structure, planning, silence, education, generosity, simplicity.... There are so many values. What has value to you may not have value to me and vice versa. This exercise is about *your* values.

Start by writing down ten values of importance to you. (If you cannot choose, then note two and write down the one that stands out for you in the moment.) Reduce your list to three that resonate right now. Then hold these, bringing some awareness of your values into contemplation daily so that they can feed this inner light. Periodically, every few months, revisit your list. How have your values changed?

Visualization

Envision your life.

How do you imagine your life three months from now?

Write one sentence for every area of your life: your feelings, thoughts, physical health, mental health, soul health; your environment; your use of time; your family, relationship, friends, wealth, and so on. Now, visualize further into the future of your life:

- How do you envision your life three years from now?

- What kind of feelings do you have? Thoughts, physical health, mental health?

- How do you envision your life ten years from now?

- How do you see your legacy?

- How do you wish to be remembered? How do you wish to have contributed to others' lives? Your family, colleagues, children, community, people known and unknown to you? Perhaps animals, oceans and waterways, the forest and land, the environment....

I invite you to do a contemplation.

There is only one light,
The great light of your own heart.
Meditate on this awareness,
"I am light. Light is me. I am light. I am"
I am born of the light.
I am composed of the light.
My very essence is light.
I am the sound of the light.
The light is my great feminine essence
The sound of my womanhood is the light.
Of the light I am.
In the light I live.
From the light I serve.
To the light I return.

Now imagine a grand vision of your life. A moment in which you can look back upon your entire life in all its wholeness. This moment is your glorious life celebration. Your friends, your family, those dearest to you are all here with you, to celebrate and honor you and all your contributions. To acknowledge all that you have given, all that you have shared, all that you have sacrificed, all your service throughout the course of your rich, blessed life.

A dear loved one is about to speak of your legacy, of what you have created in your life, how you have influenced her life as a woman. What would you deeply wish her to say of you? How do you want to be remembered? You are so safe, you are so loved, you are so precious. What would you truly wish to have her say of you? What would you really like to create in your life? Why would people be so grateful to have known you? What did you do in life through living your wisdom? What did you share? What kind of life did you live? Who did you love? Who loved you?

The people in your life are so grateful to know you. Why are they so grateful to know this magnificent wise woman who is you? This radiant woman.

Contemplate this. See it. Taste it. Touch it. Smell it. Feel it. Celebrate. Love.

You are a radiant woman. You have journeyed so courageously through life. Through your phases of life to this very moment.

You have dipped your brush into the vast realms of Ayurveda and the yoga of sound, discovering ways to create absolute vitality for how you live your life. You have many great tools to draw upon.

You can go deeper. I invite you to continue to go deeper. To continue to refine your radiance, your effulgent light.

May our feeling penetrate into the center of our hearts
And seek in love to unite itself with human beings
sharing the same goals
And with spirit beings who, bearing grace
And strengthening us from realms of light
And illuminating our love,
Are gazing down upon our earnest, heartfelt striving.
DR. RUDOLF STEINER

IV

The Resounding Design by Creation

CHAPTER 18

The Guṇas:
Qualities of Being

. . . .

WHEREAS THE DOṢAS are the governing forces of the body, the *guṇas* are the qualities of our mind. We are always looking at ways to develop more sāttvic or pure qualities, particularly the qualities of our mental channels and the mind. The guṇas are, in essence qualities, of nature.[1] "Guṇa" is Sanskrit for "what binds." When the guṇas are not correctly understood, they keep one in bondage to the external world.

There are forces all around us, within us, and throughout the entire universe: life forces, death forces, creative and destructive, positive, negative, ascending, descending, light, heavy. Some of these forces can elevate you. You can experience greater understanding, more peacefulness within yourself, within your mind and heart. Others can make you feel dull, heavy, confused, attached to things, attached to outcomes.

Essentially, the resonance and dominant qualities of these guṇas living in us by nature is known as truth and ignorance. Illumination and shadow. Light and dark. It is all inherent in us but it's about the ratios. There is a duality to this this kind of qualitative nature, which is how you navigate your way through life as you both survive and find meaning. It's about understanding and integration. This is a need common to all people, to all women.

These forces, these qualities, have currents that oppose each other. You have the task of navigating your way through them so that you can cultivate the qualities of ascending spiritual forces and not be too bound in the descending inertia that lacks spirituality. That means not thinking you are only your physical body in limited form. And, my dear one, you are so very much more.

Mother Nature is the divine mother manifesting as the play of consciousness in the universe. She gives for outward, material growth, expansion, and inward spiritual growth and development. Through nature we see these forces at play. Observing these qualities imparts understanding of the forces of the feminine essence at play, too.

And within nature is a qualitative energy. We can expand into wisdom or contract into ignorance by what dominates within us. Such qualities operate through conscious forces. They can be healing or harming. Instinctively, we know this by nature. However, many of us do not consciously remember this because so many layers and veils obscure this knowingness—hence we forget how to nurture, to cultivate these qualitative resonances. Generally, we are not taught this stuff in the school curriculum!

Pulling back the veils that cloud our perception, understanding this light and shadow, cultivating the guṇas is thus our task. This is part of an Ayurvedic woman's curriculum, part of the language of vitality.

Understanding this is fundamental to healing and working with the quality of your mind. You can understand how these qualities work in life, in the world, and within you.

According to Ayurveda, there are three primal qualities that are the main power of cosmic intelligence. These are what determine our spiritual growth. That means that having a conscious relationship to these qualities shapes how you evolve as a woman.

In the second half of life, these forces are called on to work in a more refined, qualitative way, as they are more active by nature.

The three guṇas and their qualities:

1. *Sāttva:* This guṇa's essence is intelligence; it imparts balance.

2. *Rājas:* This guṇa's essence is energy; it causes imbalance.

3. *Tāmas:* This guṇa's essence is substance; it creates inertia.

These subtle and not so subtle qualities underpin the mind, physical matter, and life. Ayurveda says that these are the powers of the soul that hold the *karma* and desires that propel us from birth to birth. Now, this is a big, imaginative picture to hold, so take it in slowly!

Everything, each object in the entire universe, is a composition of all three guṇas. We need all three qualities of the guṇas, just as we need all three governing forces, the doṣas. However, the qualities of the guṇas create a deeper level than the doṣas and are able to give us better understanding of our mental and true spiritual nature as a human being. As a woman.

Sāttva

Sāttva is the quality of intelligence that creates purity and goodness. It creates harmony, balance, inner stability, equilibrium, and equipoise. Its qualitative nature is light and luminous. It provides happiness and contentment that is established and lasting by nature. It is clarity, expansiveness, peacefulness, and the force of love that unites us.

When you are moved by the beauty of nature, a flower, a bird, the rising sun, just for what it is, this is sāttvic. Mother Teresa was sāttvic. She served for the highest purpose, to simply be of service without attachment, from a place of purity.

Rājas

Rājas is the quality of activity, change, turbulence. It introduces disharmony and disequilibrium that upsets existing balance. Rājas is motivated, driven in action, ever seeking, and goal orientated, which is what gives it power.

Rājas has an outward motion that makes it external and uses self-seeking action that ultimately leads to fragmentation and dissolution. It is stimulating and gives pleasure but only in the short term. Its destabilizing nature means that it results in pain and suffering. Rājas is a force of passion that can ultimately lead to conflict and distress.

When I really, really want that new pair of boots, I am dominated by rājas. The pleasure that they bring is short-lived. They do not fit any more or they fall apart, or they are no longer exotic or stylish in my eyes. Or they may be totally impractical. This is an illustration of rājas.

Tāmas

Tāmas is the quality of inertia, dullness, darkness. Heavy by nature, it veils, covers, and obstructs. It blocks. It works like the force of gravity that holds things in a limited form. It retards growth. Tāmas has a downward motion that causes decay and disintegration. Tāmas brings ignorance and can bring delusion. It encourages sleepiness within you. Tāmas dulls awareness and it desensitizes. Tāmas is the principle of unconsciousness or materiality that veils your true nature and understanding.

The Three Guṇas Together

We need all three of these qualities. For example, to build a house, there has to be an impulse, a vision of pure imagination. This is the spark of motion to start. Rājas is the drive, the force, the motivation and passion to get the house built. Tāmas is what brings closure to the house. It installs the doors, roof, walls and brings boundaries to limit the form of the house, which would otherwise keep growing and growing.

If the vision were purely sāttvic, it could become ever-grander but the house may never be built of bricks and mortar. And without the tāmas it would not come to completion.

We need all three, but we strive for more illumination and sāttvic quality. Sāttva creates the clarity of mind through which we perceive the truth of things as they are, as we are. It gives light, concentration, pure imagination, devotion. And, dear woman, devotion to the self is what lands you at the feet of the divine. The mind is by nature the domain of sāttva.

Rājas and tāmas, however, are the points of mental disharmony, confusion, agitation, irritation, and delusion. They bring about incorrect imagination or lack of truthful perception. They can bring false understanding of the external world as it really is and are a cause of seeking happiness and joy outside of yourself, losing inner equilibrium and connection, thinking that if you have what you see around you it will bring happiness, fulfillment, purpose, and accomplishment. This is prevalent in the modern world, an external, material world. Desire, turbulence, and emotional upset are all created by rājas.

This seeking to fulfill desires is different than indulging oneself from a place of celebration, where you enjoy the chocolate as an expression of life rather than eat it because you think it will fill a deep need that is wanting. This is why it's important do inner reflection and have repose, to cultivate a more sāttvic quality of your being.

Tāmas brings ignorance of your true nature. It creates veils and thus it weakens your power of clear perception, leading to confusion and uncertainty. It keeps you second-guessing yourself. These veils can create separation of self, which can be isolating and lead to depression.

Tāmas is prevalent in consciousness that is identified with the physical body. If this is all you think you are, then this is dull. Tāmas resonates heavily and is so very limited. When you identify yourself with the physical only, you remain in the realm of tāmas influence.

Even sāttva is balanced by rājas and tāmas. They give energy and stability. Otherwise, you'd float away. You would not be able to function effectively in the world.

However, sāttva as a state of harmony is responsible for healing and health. Your vitality is maintained by sāttvic living, which is existing harmoniously with nature and with yourself. Looking after your inner garden, cultivating qualities of purity, clarity, peacefulness in order to nurture the virtue of love.

Rājas and tāmas are causative factors of disease. Rājas causes pain and agitation, dissipation and dissolving of your vital life energy— particularly for a woman in the second half of life.

Tāmas brings stagnation, decay, and death processes. They usually work together. Rājas is seen as overexerting expression and energy, which depletes and leads to fatigue. The destabilizing aspect of its nature means it's simply not sustainable. For example, if you have too much stimulating activity, too much exercise or external activity, food, alcohol, or sex, over time these lead to fatigue and dullness. Too much rājas or turbulent emotions drives mental stimulation at first and leads to mental dullness, depression, and the exhaustion of life forces.

For vitality and radiance and for a meaningful life, a healthy, creative, spiritual life, we strive for more sāttvic qualities. You possess a quality of mind, a clarity that cuts off the psychological root of disease. You can see meaning in life, life experiences, and challenges, in both joy and pain. Life is seen as a rich learning experience and with appreciation and gratitude you look for the good in all situations, even loss, grief, and disease. There's essentially a striving to understand, for integration, and to constantly build this muscle of resilience instead of suppressing and putting bandages over wounds and hurts.

Cultivate Sāttvic Qualities
· ·

When we work with the guṇas therapeutically, we are working with the quality of light. Let's then look at ways to cultivate more sāttvic guṇa.

The first stage is always to break up tāmas and develop rājas. There needs to be an activation to create energy, to stimulate, and to break up that which is dull and inert. That means moving from mental inertia and stagnation to self-driven action.

The second stage is to pacify and calm rājas and develop more sāttva. We move from self-motivated action to selfless service and right action.

The final stage is moving from selfless service to a state of meditation, moving from ignorance and physically oriented living to vitality and self-expression, to peace and illumination.

Ayurvedically, this is how we work, and all tools, practices, remedies, and therapies follow this pathway of working qualitatively. In short, we stimulate tāmas, motivate rājas, and cultivate sāttva.

In Ayurveda, we encourage a vegetarian or more plant-based diet, meditation, and mantra in order to break up the tāmas and create more lightness. Mantra is very powerful for cultivating sāttva in the mental channels, as it breaks up heaviness and dullness.

The right kind of warmth in the organism is needed here. Fire is required to burn the dross away from the gold. Warmth, energy, and activity are generated by the fire to create change. This fire awakens one to the potential and impulse to create transformation. Here, deep-seated patterns of attachment, habits, depression, stagnation, and procrastination are let go. They are mobilized and released. You can actually let go of habits. Typically, this calls you to really look at yourself. Recognize, confront your pain and suffering, and look at where you have suppressed pain, lack, and hurts for years. It's not only recognizing but also learning from the task of your pain. The ability is created to let go of the that story you've created and told yourself repeatedly, which has become boring. Year after year of telling the same story has embedded it deeper into your patterning. When working with the guṇas, you have the potential to shape-shift, to change the story that you strongly identify with, to create a new story of what you wish to become. It is a wonderful thing to cultivate more of this quality in your life.

When you do this, you are still vulnerable to the pains, challenges, and hurts of life. However, you can experience your problems in a new way and make them a little less personal. You can understand a little more about yourself, the human condition, and the hurts and needs of all people, and thus experience life with a little more detachment. You can connect with others with greater compassion. It makes you more charitable in the truest sense. You can take more action and do things from a place of service, being more in touch with your life's purpose on a spiritual level. This is the key to your vitality and your radiance.

This is why we meditate: to create inner space, a space to observe, to listen, to be divinely inspired. You watch what comes up and allow it to move through you in meditation, and you have the space to let it go. Meditation cultivates inner stillness and quietude.

Here is a mantra for abundance, prosperity, deep beauty, and vitality—an abundance of ojas. I work with this mantra therapeutically for clients to become embedded in their vitality.

Auṁ Hrīṁ Śrīṁ Klīṁ Mahālakṣmyai Namaḥ
(pronounced *"aum hreem shreem kleem*
mahaa lakshmayaye namaha")

Enrichment Activity #9 in appendix F includes a chart showing how mental qualities relate to the guṇas. I encourage you to complete this chart. It is not an exercise in having the purest qualities. There are no right or wrong answers. There are only authentic answers, which can then support you. I thus invite you to be authentic and honest when you complete this exercise. You may wish to have a friend or partner complete it with you because somebody who knows you intimately will most likely be more objective about you than you are about yourself.

When I first completed this chart with a buddy, we really wanted to be pure and were ticking off the boxes to reflect that. A third person present, a very solid German Ayurvedic therapist and divine woman, said, "You know, we are all a lot more tāmasic than we'd like to think we are." We laughed and got real! We started again and ticked the boxes more authentically, which revealed more truly the qualities we possessed at that time.

Because you change, do this exercise a few times a year. It's a revealing way to check in with the state of your mind. Have fun with this check-in. Get into the weed pulling of your inner garden. And if you are dwelling inwardly in a divine abundant food forest, then share the fruits of this with other women and daughters.

We need to have a new impulse, an aliveness to who we are and what we need to do. Action is necessary—rājas. Not only action in the mind but in the outer aspects of our lives. That can look so different for everyone. It may be as simple as getting out of bed, getting off the couch in front of the TV, and moving your body. Getting out in nature. Getting into the daylight. Going for a walk. So this stage is one of breaking up, mobilizing, modifying, allowing in new potential.

When we are softening, pacifying rājas and cultivating more sāttva, we need spaciousness. This is why repose is so necessary for your inner growth, development, and authenticity. Yoga is wonderful because it offers an opportunity to create inner spaciousness. It's not about doing lots of headstands and physically twisting yourself into a knot; it's about working with your mental channels—a union between mind and body.

When we meditate we create an inner spaciousness. We observe. We watch what comes up and allow it to move through us. We create space to release. We create space to listen. We create space to be divinely inspired.

The spaciousness is required because without it we cannot surrender. What are we surrendering? When we cultivate more sāttvic qualities we are surrendering our attachments: to our pain, our ways of thinking that create our suffering, our attachment to that very suffering, our attachment to our stories. We are releasing the grip on all our hurts and pet peeves, all the things that have been done to us, how we've been wronged. We are forgiving.

In the greater picture, we're surrendering our personal, ego-driven agendas, desires, and personal motivation for that of a greater cause, which is healing and of benefit to humanity. We cultivate service, and service born of such impulse gives vitality.

It's not that we don't have problems, hurts, or pains anymore. We do but we are able to make them a bit less personal and understand a bit more the human condition and hurts of all people. We connect with others and their problems with more compassion and empathy. It is charitable. It is service, and it's inner evolution and development on a spiritual level. This is the task of your life. This is the key to your vitality, and so we strive to cultivate qualities that are more sāttvic.

Many of you have been doing this for years and I'm just explaining what you are doing from an Ayurvedic perspective and how you are cultivating these pure qualities of harmony. This is the core and essential teaching of Ayurvedic philosophy.

CHAPTER 19

Manifestations of Karma

. . . .

KARMA IS A vast subject whose laws encompass the very mysteries of existence. "Karma" literally means "action." There is a tendency to think of karma as associated with good or bad. But karma in itself is neutral. It is a law of action and reaction.

There is literally no escaping your karma in life. However, you can change how you perceive your karma. You can work with the lessons of it and, in so doing, peel through the many veils of ignorance, revealing your truth.

As a law of cause and effect, or action–reaction, it is important to develop karmic awareness as a vehicle in which you journey through your life.

As life is rhythm in motion, there is a constancy of movement, and this means the law of karma, too, is always manifesting action–reaction.

Karmic awareness allows us to unlock the karmic merry-go-round so that we can evolve as conscious women. We can attain a greater capability for individual freedom in the choices we make from moment to moment.

For me, understanding karma makes it easier to navigate life and to mind my own business!

It gives me greater capacity to accept how it can be that people have such extremely different experiences, events, and circumstances to deal with in their lives, even the meaning of disease, health, and illness, the curable and incurable, and accidents and natural disasters. As a woman, as a mother, as a human being, I find this helpful in accepting, trusting, and surrendering. Developing a comprehension of karma as a real scientific phenomenon can provide answers to life's mysterious questions as we seek meaning.

Dr. Rudolf Steiner, in his book *Manifestations of Karma*, notes, "We create our own karma in all areas of existence, laying the foundation in one incarnation for the following one. We cannot seek for a complete pattern or meaning in one earthly life but must begin to consider many lives on Earth. Although we may not always be aware of the particular causes of events, know that we are resolving our own self-induced karma can help to bring both an acceptance and a sense of purpose of our lives."

As we start to develop greater awareness of how karma works, how our personal karma is interwoven with that of groups, communities of people, and all humanity is revealed. This means that, as we ponder the law of karma, we are able to raise our conscious awareness about the vital role we play in how we contribute, or don't, to serve worldly evolution.

CHAPTER 20

Your Sound, Your Song

Music melts all the separate parts of our bodies together.
ANAÏS NIN

Mantra Puruṣa

In addition to our gross physical body, our flesh and bones, our nerves and blood, skin and hair, the body we so strongly and consciously identify with is another subtle body.

This subtle body is our sound body. It is an energy body that is composed of the resonance of sound. And yoga says that our higher self is connected to our physical body through this body of sound.

This is why sound is yoga. The yoga of sound. *Nāda* yoga.

When the yogi is absorbed in the nāda,
the external world falls away and bliss arises.
ŚIVA SAṂHITĀ, 5.45

This yoga of mantra, of sound, has the capacity to teach us how to harmonize our own subtle body of sound to create the right flow of energy in our physical body, and in our mental channels of the mind.

Mantra comes from the words *manas*, meaning the mind, and *tra*, to protect. A mantra is that which protects the mind.

A mantra is a collection of syllables and letters that have a penetrating, activating resonance that can break up dullness, stagnation, blockage, and that which keeps you bound in thought, feeling, limitation, and contraction.[2]

Mantra syllables and sounds can penetrate and awaken subtle, refined activity of the mind while pacifying and nourishing the nervous system.

Mantra is a tool for penetrating our limited perception, thoughts, habits, and patterns. We can use it to hang on in times of great challenge, resistance, fear, and overwhelm. We can use it to transcend, transmute, and transform our lives.

Mantra is to the mind what yoga āsana is to the physical body. Hence mantra as yoga. And, when practicing with one-pointed focus, listening awareness, and discernment, mantra is āsana practice in itself, fully working each cell, tissue, diaphragm, and organ of our bodies.

With correct placement of Sanskrit sounds, mantra can dissolve resistance and limitations. That means it annihilates fear and contraction, leaving expansion, light, and love.

It is for this very reason that great teachers, spiritual leaders, and wise beings use mantra and encourage japa, the practice of the repetition of mantra.

Sanskrit is called the "universal language" and "the language of the Gods." Dr. David Frawley says that this is no mere exaggeration because Sanskrit reflects the primal sounds of creation. These sounds are embodied in the letters of the Sanskrit alphabet.

Hence, the Sanskrit alphabet is more than just a group of sounds. From the perspective of tantra, it's the creative play of consciousness into form. When we directly experience the sounds, they come alive.

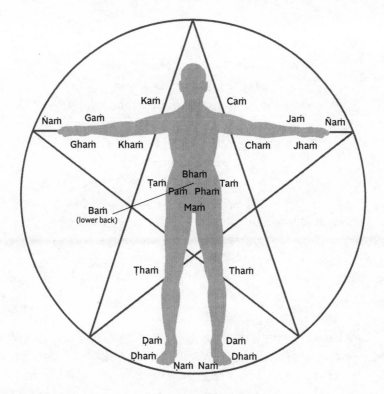

Now, this is mystical, but we actually have the experience of mantra, of the sounds as an enlivened harmonizing dynamic.

Sanskrit is a language of cosmic vibration and sound. The very vibrations of the cosmos are contained in the sounds of each letter of the Sanskrit alphabet. Each letter of the Sanskrit alphabet corresponds to a particular area of the physical body. This is what we know as *mantra puruṣa*. It is literally the cosmic person made of mantra.

Mantra puruṣa can create the quality of illumination. This is the quality of light. The classic philosophical book *A Course in Miracles* says that only the mind is capable of illumination. The spirit is already illuminated. The physical body itself is too dense. However, the mind can bring its illumination to the body. Mantra practice works on the quality of the mind. And the body can come into alignment when the mind has the quality that looks beyond identification with only the body to this very light.

Through mantra you can heal the sound
pattern of your entire being.
Letting the mantra take over for the agitation
of your thoughts and bring wholeness and
equipoise to your entire nature.
DR. DAVID FRAWLEY

Practicing mantra puruṣa daily is like sonically cleaning all your channels, tissues, and body parts. It is a spiritual hygiene practice. When you chant, you are sweeping inner pathways so that processes and flow can be optimal. The sheaths that compose your breath, your awareness, your thoughts, your vitality are all sonically cleansed when you bring your awareness to each body part and your tissues as your chant mantra puruṣa.

You can chant the mantra puruṣa daily, bringing your focus to each body part area, perhaps pointing lightly to each with your fingers. If you know the Sanskrit alphabet, you can include the bīja, or seed letter sound. For beginners, I recommend bringing your focus to the body part and chanting "auṁ," "auṁ aiṁ," or "auṁ hrīṁ śrīṁ."

Mantra puruṣa not only affects the physical body. The subtle body of sound vibrations also relates to the mental body, the astral or feeling body, and cakras, or major energy centers.

In working with the frequencies and resonance of this sound body, you can create healing of the body and the quality of your mind. This is why it's a deeply penetrating tool of mantra used in Ayurvedic medicine. And, like all tools, the more skilled you become at using it, the more refined and penetrating it becomes.

Hence, I encourage you to cultivate a practice of reciting the mantra puruṣa daily.

You can do this by either chanting an auṁ and bringing your consciousness, prāṇa, and listening awareness to this body part and tissue as described in the subtle body map.

To establish yourself in the experience of the mantra puruṣa, I recommend doing a forty-day practice. Each and every day, consecutively for forty days, chant the mantra puruṣa. If you miss a day, start again at day one. Doing this as a forty-day practice will establish you in the beneficial qualitative experience it generates. Although any time of day is suitable, I recommend first thing in the morning, as part of an inner contemplative practice.

> Upon the rhythm of the breath health depends.
> This at once shows that both the
> mind and body are sound when musical,
> and disorderly when unmusical.
> **HAZRAT INAYAT KHAN**

Bīja (Seed Sounds)

Seed sounds, or bīja mantras, are primary combinations of single syllables of the Sanskrit alphabet.

They are sound combinations of elemental alphabet sounds. These sounds are representative of elements, atoms, chemical processes coming together to create particular qualities.

These seed sounds, when repeated as mantra, can impart inner experiences that correlate to the distinct qualities of the bīja. For example, *yaṁ*. This sound brings juiciness to your being, nourishing your heart forces, your plasma, lymph, and flavor for life. It is a sound that nourishes your vitality, or ojas.

By taking each letter and adding an "ṁ" to it, you turn that letter into a bīja mantra. The effect of this is more meditative, as this "ṁ" is an *anusvāra*. This means it is an after-sound that follows a vowel, or a dissolving inward sound.

The "ṁ" sound is made by bringing the lips together and then ever so lightly touching the roof of the mouth with the tip of your tongue. Try making this sound (*mmmmm*) just with your lips together and tongue resting on the lower palate behind your bottom teeth. Then try again with the tip of your tongue touching the roof of your mouth. Switch between these positions several times and feel the difference. It's subtle but listen into this feeling. Why? Because you are working with sonic sound and to have the full potential of its healing effect, you must experience it.

You can use the practice of mantra puruṣa to work with the quality of your vitality, the quality of your mind, the quality of the tissues, including your plasma, lymph, blood, nerve, bone, and fat. You can use the mantra to bring the right flow into all channels of communication in your body, from the grossest to the subtlest. Thus, this mantra is used to create your own healing and wellness. Just as you know you must sweep the inner path clean regularly through cleansing and right lifestyle, you also know that routine and regularity support your inner rhythms. You are composed of rhythm, and mantra is the resonance and sound of this very rhythm.

Chanting is a significant and mysterious practice. It is the highest nectar, a tonic that fully nourishes our inner being. Chanting opens the heart and makes love flow within us. It releases such intoxicating inner bliss and enthusiastic splendor, that simply through the nectar it generates, we can enter the abode of the Self.
SWAMI MUKTANANDA

In the Sanskrit alphabet are groups of sounds in fifty letters. These are vowels, consonants, semivowels, and sibilants. These sets of sounds relate to regions of the body:

- **Vowels:** Sixteen vowels relate to the head and senses.

- **Consonants:** Twenty-five consonants relate to the joints of arms and legs (including hips), abdomen, navel, and lower back.

- **Semivowels and sibilants:** Nine semivowels and sibilants relate to the seven levels of tissues, or dhātus, and primary components of the entire body from the lymph to the prāṇa and mind.

These are the letters of the Sanskrit alphabet as they relate to each area of the body:

VOWELS: HEAD AND ORGANS OF SENSE

A	top of head	Ḷ	right cheek
Ā	forehead	Ḹ	left cheek
I	right eye	E	upper lip
Ī	left eye	AI	lower lip
U	right ear	O	upper teeth
Ū	left ear	AU	lower teeth
R	right nostril	Ṁ	upper palate
Ṝ	left nostril	Ḥ	lower palate

CONSONANTS: LIMBS, NAVEL, AND ABDOMEN

K	right shoulder	Ṭ	right hip
KH	right elbow	ṬH	right knee
G	right wrist	Ḍ	right ankle
GH	right base fingers	ḌH	right base toes
Ṅ	right tips fingers	Ṇ	right tips toes
C	left shoulder	T	left hip
CH	left elbow	TH	left knee
J	left wrist	D	left ankle
JH	left base fingers	DH	left base toes
Ñ	left tips fingers	N	left tips toes
P	right abdomen		
PH	left abdomen		
B	lower back		
BH	navel		
M	lower belly		

SEMIVOWELS AND SIBILANTS: DHĀTUS (BODY TISSUES)

Y	rasa (plasma and lymph)	Ś	asthi (bone)
R	rakta (blood)	Ṣ	majja (nerve tissue, marrow)
L	māmsa (muscle)	S	śukra (reproductive)
V	medha (fat)	H	prāṇa (soul)
		KṢ	mind

Before its incarnation the soul is sound.
It is for this reason that we love sound.
HAZRAT INAYAT KHAN

Sound as Your Medicine

Sound is the essence and very composition of all matter in the universe. It is patterns and sequences of vibrations that give form to substance. Sound is applicable to everything in nature, and to you as a woman.

Dr. Claudia Welch says that when you live a life of balance, your hormones become balanced. As long as there is stress in your being, your hormones cannot be in full balance. It is my belief that we are able to bring our entire being and lives into balance when we listen deeply into our own sound. Sound is medicine for our thoughts that have an immediate effect on our physiology. And our thoughts have a much more immediate and penetrating effect on our physiology than food.

The source of sound is from a vast realm of the cosmos where spirit resides. The patterns of all sounds have a rhythm. It is for this reason that nature is rhythmical. This, too, is why all the seasons and cycles of nature, along with all our human biological patterns, are rhythmical in shade and tone. This applies to the sacred rhythms of womankind, the rhythms of the menstrual cycle, and the rhythms of the great mother.

Intrinsically, we are rhythmical, musical beings.

**Since every night during sleep man's soul lives in the spiritual
world—essentially a light-filled ocean of sounds—
it is understandable why music speaks so directly and
powerfully to almost everyone.**
DR. RUDOLF STEINER

In music, the melodies of tones are a direct expression of the sounds of nature. Dr. Rudolf Steiner says the musician hears the pulse of the divine will that flows through the world, hears how this will expresses itself in tones. The musician thus stands closer to the heart of the world than all other artists. Since music flows nearer the heart of the world and is a direct expression of its surging and swelling, it also directly affects the human soul. This gives us an imaginative picture of how the effects of music on the human soul are direct, penetrating, powerful, and elemental.

These rhythms that exist in each and every process of your body are to be cared for in a holistic approach, in order to remain vital in all aspects of your wellness. Take, for example, the role of the spleen. This vital organ plays a significant role in maintaining health through its relationship to rhythm. The function of the spleen is to harmonize the ultimate and inevitable effects of your lifestyle on the rhythm of your digestive process. It regulates discrepancies and irregularities that constantly appear in the rhythmic processes of digestion. It monitors and communicates these discrepancies to your liver that can then discern and enliven, again in a rhythmical way, our blood. Curiously, too much thinking, over time, can deplete and disrupt the rhythms of this compassionate organ.

Sound becomes visible in the form of radiance in the physical body. In this way, the physical absorbs the energy of sound and becomes charged with new magnetism.

Music in the soul can be heard by the Universe.
LAO TZU

Everyone is gifted with a unique pitch from God, the natural note of each person. If practiced, if refined and cared for, this pitch develops qualitatively. The sound of your being, of your voice both heard and unheard has a resonance and a rhythm that are miraculous and healing. It is your radiance.

The Yoga of Sound

Nāda yoga is the yoga of sound. It's a yoga of listening to the inner streaming of sound, and literally means union or yoking through sound. Given that sound is the substance of all matter of the universe, what a wonderful thing to yoke with! Although nāda yoga is a musical practice, typically it is an inward-focused practice used as a tool for your own transformation and not external for performance.

Nāda yoga is ancient like Ayurveda. It dates back more than four thousand years to the *Rig Veda*, one of the world's oldest-known classic spiritual texts. It teaches about meditation on nāda, the inner sacred sound.

The practices of nāda yoga employ the ancient tools of this art and spiritual science as meditation on sound. Nāda yoga is a path to realization of the self. It is an autonomous self-practice accessible and appropriate for all people of any age, caste, creed, religion, or spiritual orientation.

Sound is a penetrating and empowering form of yoga because it is effortless for our minds to become absorbed in it. If you watch infants, children, the elderly, and people of varying ages in between, you see that we take pleasure in listening to music. Animals, too, enjoy the sound of music.

Anandra George, founder of Heart of Sound, the world's first yoga teacher training based on nāda yoga, says, "When the mind is fully concentrated on anything, there arises a feeling of inner bliss. In nāda yoga, we learn that the source of the sound may be external or internal, gross or subtle."

The practice of nāda yoga ultimately refines and cultivates your awareness of listening. Discernment of listening is developed, and the "sounds behind the audible sound" can start to be heard and understood. My dear woman, you can truly get to know your own nature and source. The more enlivened your listening becomes, the more of the sacred you experience in the sound.

This is purely an experiential practice. It cannot be understood or known in theory. It is a practice you simply have to do, through mantra, vocal toning, or other chanting.

About Ritual

Ritual is a set of fixed actions, and sometimes words, performed regularly, especially as part of a ceremony.

Often associated with religious ceremony, ritual is something performed regularly as part of ceremony, which imparts a quality of the sacred.

Ritual is rich and infused with meaning. Ritual, when done with reverence and awareness, can be a divine act of self-love. In this way ritual can impart true radiance to your very being.

Conclusion

· · · · · · · · · · · ·

A GOLDEN THREAD weaves its way throughout the very being of the Ayurvedic woman.

This thread is composed of consciousness. This thread is what pulsates throughout your entire being. It weaves all your experiences from moment to moment, year to year, decade to decade, even life to life. It is what you bring with you. It is all you take with you.

Our tāmasic tendencies dull the resonance of the thread. They block the golden light that is produced from the reverberation of this very thread. This is because tāmas is too heavy for the light to penetrate, and that's exactly how we become bound by inertia and ignorance when we have too much of it.

Aam too blocks the path and fullness of this illuminating resonance. When this happens, it means your radiance is dimmed.

A musician would never play her stringed instrument without first tuning it. Listening with awareness to the pitch, the sound, the resonance until it reverberated sweetly in her whole being. A musician cares for her instrument. Constantly adjusting the tension of the strings, putting resin on the bow. Feeling into, breathing into the sound of the instrument. Merging with the instrument, becoming the doing, not being the doer.

When you work with sound tools, when you work with mantra, the penetration of the resonance is able to activate, mobile, break up the tamas, the dullness, the stinky sludge that keeps you bound and limited. The fire of the sound transmutes into action and then refines, purifies and illumines. You are tuning your instrument and allowing the sound of your divinity to play through you.

It takes great effort to pass through the eye of the needle. Great discipline and focus are required. It can feel difficult beyond words. However, it is through the very eye of the needle that this golden thread must go in order to expand into the love that is your very nature, to expand into the great feminine you are. Dear woman, benevolent grace is what follows your efforts. It sits in full splendor awaiting you on the other side of your effort.

May you remember your way as a divine soul in the body and image of woman. May your life be full of ritual that gives meaning, purpose, and radiance to all that you are.

Acknowledgments

· · · · · · · · · · · ·

I ACKNOWLEDGE WITH immense love my family. They have made great sacrifice that I may pursue what calls me to be in loving service and contribution in the writing of this book. Graeme, Jake, Callum, Rumi, Luca, and Tamar: I could not be who I am without your teaching and love. Graeme, your constancy, tenacity, all-embracing encouragement and belief in me to write are the greatest blessing.

I acknowledge my grandmothers, my mother, my sister and my beloved daughters.

Enormous thanks to all the loving and unwaveringly supportive, enthusiastic team at Page Two. Orchestrating, guiding, editing, designing, and keeping me on task.

Thanks to Geoff Affleck for being such a supporter and always being so generous and available for me.

I also acknowledge all you great beings in all realms who believe in me and support me unwaveringly. You each know who you are. I love you.

I've had the great privilege of wonderful teachers and mentors who have believed in me, taught, guided, and encouraged me in mysterious, profound, deeply meaningful ways.

To Dr. Pankaj Naram for teaching me the art of pulse reading. Dr. Smita Naram for your guidance, sisterhood, divine feminine, and revered friendship. Irmhild Kleinhenz for always acknowledging all I know, allowing me to deepen my love and wisdom of Ayurveda while expanding my love of healing mysteries and the human in anthroposophical medicine. And to Anandra George, for your teaching, friendship, and the opportunity to refine, grow, and expand in the resonance of sound.

To Dr. Rudolf Steiner for the gift of anthroposophy and Dr. Ita Wegman for anthroposophical medicine I give immeasurable gratitude and love for the impulse to renew ancient healing mysteries.

I acknowledge all women. Women of past, women of present, women of future.

To my beloved Guru. SGMKJ.

Cleansing

. . . .

Effective Aam-Reducing Practices

To reduce aam, Ayurveda recommends the following:

- The most effective home practice to cleanse tissue and reduce aam is to fast with mung soup. The duration of the fast depends on the level of aam in the tissue. The most gentle and regular way to cleanse with mung soup is to do so one day a week. For a deeper cleanse, try three consecutive days each month. For an even deeper, penetrating experience, do a seven-day cleanse annually.

- On the cleanse days, eat only mung soup. Eat as much as you need but only this food. To end the seven-day mono-food fast, add cooked vegetables like pumpkin, squash, zucchini, sweet potato, and leafy greens to your diet for two days. Add rice on the third day after the cleanse. Gently return to your regular diet, reintroducing foods gradually. Doing a seven-day mung cleanse requires more planning and preparation to be ready and committed to it. However, it is penetrating, cleansing, and recalibrating in profound ways and absolutely worth the effort!

- If you are feeling heavy in the gut or have eaten something that is rich and heavy, the antidote to this feeling is eating mung soup as the next meal or fasting on it for half a day.

- Drink ginger tea regularly.

- Take half a teaspoon of ginger juice with a teaspoon of honey twice daily.

The Recalibrate Cleanse

The Recalibrate Cleanse is, in essence, a deeper version of the magical mung soup day (see chapter 11, and the recipe in appendix C on page 195). The duration of this cleanse is three days. It takes mental grit and preparation to do this cleanse. If you have a social celebration then ask yourself, "Is this the kindest time for me to do this?" If you are traveling, have house guests, if it's Thanksgiving, Easter, or whatever celebration it may be on the calendar, then it may not be the three days most conducive to cleansing. Be strategic in the most loving way to really support yourself to do this cleanse with gentleness and ease. Do you drink coffee and have deadlines to meet? These are all the things to consider with timing. Although, if you are heading into great demands and challenges, the clarity and focus you will get from cleansing is wonderful. And the lightness of your digestive load makes tasks much easier on the body during really busy times. Experiment, and try it on for yourself.

Be prepared. Have your ingredients on hand to make the soup, because on the first day, when you have mung soup for breakfast, unless the pot is on simmer you'll be hungry.

For this three-day cleanse, start each day by sipping on one teaspoon of ghee mixed in hot water.

Eat only mung soup. Make sure the soup has a broth-like consistency, with plenty of liquid, not thick like dal.

You can have as much soup as you like, but eat only mung soup for these three days.

Drink ginger tea between meals. You can also drink the metabolic spice tea (see recipe in appendix C on page 197).

Take one teaspoon of vaca oil, or castor oil, before bed.

Keep a journal during these three days, dedicating ten minutes (yes, just ten sacred minutes!) daily to writing whatever comes to you. All you have to do is show up with intention, attention, ease, pen, and journal. The words will come. You may like to kick things off by writing about what you are grateful for, or perhaps for what you are feeling, even needing.

The Seven-Day Radiance Mung Cleanse

DAYS ONE TO THREE
Follow the steps in the three-day Recalibrate Cleanse.

Days Four to Seven

As with days one to three, start each day with one teaspoon of ghee mixed in hot water and eat only mung soup. However, you can now add vegetables to the soup or eat veggies separately. Veggies can include pumpkin, sweet potato, zucchini, broccoli, spinach, chard (silver beet), parsnips, turnips, beetroot, carrots, or celery.

Continue taking one teaspoon of vaca oil, or castor oil, before bed. Plus take three Ayushakti Virechan tablets before bed.

On night seven, take six Ayushakti Virechan tablets before bed.

Throughout the cleanse, you can drink ginger tea and herbal teas.

General Ayurvedic Diet Guidelines for Woman's Radiance

. . . .

IN THE AYURVEDIC tradition, certain principles apply to a diet that promotes health, strength, luster, and connectedness for all phases of life, including when, where, and how foods are to be eaten.

I recommend following these principles for when, where, and how foods are eaten:

- Say a prayer or blessing on your food, acknowledging the sacred source of your food.

- Ideally eat your meals in a quiet, relaxed environment, conducive to focusing on your food (as opposed to juggling your breakfast on your lap, negotiating your way through heavy traffic, or while running kids to soccer training or dance class). Quietude while eating supports the digestion of your food. Avoiding talking while eating allows you to concentrate on chewing. This activates the digestive enzymes, which are mixed with your food while chewing.

- Eating when at ease and calm supports digestion. When emotionally distressed, anxious or angry, it is difficult to digest your food on top of your feelings.

These are general dietary guidelines. Ojas is the subtle product of perfect digestion. It is the essence that makes each nourished cell of the body feel happiness. Diet is our own natural pharmacopoeia to maintain well-being. Food is nourishment of life. Enjoy your food.

The Basic Principles of Eating for Good Health

There are several basic principles of eating for good health:

- Cooked food is easier to digest than raw.

- Warm, soupy meals are lighter and more digestible than heavy, dry, solid foods.

- Only eat when hungry and when the previous meal has been digested.

- Eat meals at regular times of the day.

- Do not eat large meals late at night and leave two hours after eating before going to bed.

- Eat moderate amounts of food, leaving room in stomach for digestion.

- Eat food that has been freshly prepared as often as possible. Avoid leftover food that is more than twenty-four hours old. But leftovers are preferred to takeaway or fast foods.

- Eat local, organic, seasonal food whenever possible.

- Do not mix milk with honey, fruit, or fish (for example, in tuna casserole).

- Do not cook with honey. Once heated, honey becomes toxic to the body, as it sticks to the tissues.

- Avoid ice-cold foods and drinks.

- To avoid diluting the digestive juices (agni), preferably drink ten minutes before or a half an hour after a meal.

- Take ghee on a daily basis as part of your diet. Three to five teaspoons is a recommended amount of ghee to consume daily, as it balances pitta and vata, and stimulates agni, your digestive fire. Ghee imparts strength and pacifies the mental channels, calming the mind. It makes things flow the way they ought to flow!

When you become imbalanced, it may be necessary to avoid certain foods. A simple example is, if you have a fever, avoid milk, as this food feeds fever. If you have headache, avoid citrus fruit and tomato, as these will create more heat and inflammation. If you are constipated, eat fewer drying and heavy foods, such as raw salads, and avoid excessive amounts of bread.

Foods to Enjoy Regularly

WHOLE GRAINS

Basmati rice, oats, rye, spelt, quinoa, barley, buckwheat, amaranth, and polenta. Flours made from the above grains are also fine. Instead of wheat pasta, take more rice, corn, veggie, buckwheat, or quinoa noodles.

Porridge made without milk, but with cinnamon, cardamom, soaked raisins or stewed fruit, and small amounts of nuts and seeds (for example, ground linseed or sunflower). This makes an ideal breakfast. It is easy to digest, nutritious, warming, and energizing. You can add warmed milk (unhomogenized cow's milk, rice, oat, almond, or non-GMO soy).

Bread. This should mainly be eaten when toasted. The dry heat stops further fermentation. Add ghee or an unctuous spread (avocado, tahini, or butter in moderation).

VEGETABLES

Cooked vegetables such as pumpkin, sweet potato, squash, marrow/zucchini, spinach, leafy green veggies, green beans, asparagus, fennel, rutabaga, turnip, sweet corn, cooked onions, carrots, parsnips, celery, chicory, leeks, peas, snow peas, endive, rocket, avocado, and broccoli.

Lettuce, salad leaves, and sprouts are best taken at lunch, preceding the meal and served with oil. Raw vegetables such as carrots, grated beetroot, cucumber, radishes, and capsicum peppers (especially red) are best eaten minimally or avoided.

PULSES

Mung beans and split mung dal, adzuki beans, tur (toor) dal, urad (black gram) dal, and red lentils. These are easy to digest, nourishing, and balancing to the body and mind. Pulses are best soaked first and cooked to soft consistency. Always cook them with pinch asafetida to reduce gas. To get optimum nourishment from pulses, eat them with grains (especially rice or barley). Kichadi is an easy to digest, nourishing stew of rice and beans.

FRUITS

All sweet fruits, such as pears, apples, apricots, peaches, nectarines, purple grapes, cherries, sweet plums and berries, fresh figs, melons, sweet oranges, mandarins, pomegranates, mangoes, papayas, and coconuts. Bananas, which are cold in energy, are best eaten cooked. Dates, raisins, and dried fruits that don't contain sulfur are fine but best when soaked or made into a stew or porridge.

SEEDS AND NUTS

Sesame, poppy, pumpkin, and sunflower seeds. Pine nuts, almonds (without skins), walnuts, hazelnuts, and pistachios should be eaten only in small amounts, as they are heavy to digest and increase vata. Nuts are a rejuvenating food. They give strength and energy and are best soaked and made into a paste or milk. Dry-roasting nuts and seeds makes them lighter to digest. Tahini is very nutritious; high in vitamin E, calcium, and protein, it can be used in a dressing or as a spread. It is hot in nature and should be used moderately. The flesh, milk, cream, and flakes of coconuts can be used liberally.

DAIRY

Ghee. Of all dairy products ghee (clarified butter) is the best—it is like a medicine, highly pitta reducing and also vata pacifying. It can be cooked with and added to all foods. It is light and easy to digest.

Butter is to be enjoyed moderately and is better than using margarines.

Milk is a rejuvenating food that also builds tissues; this is due to its heavy, damp, cold nature. It is only to be taken warm and preferably spiced with ginger, cardamom, cinnamon, or turmeric to counteract its cold, damp, and heavy qualities. If using cow's milk, only use unhomogenized milk. Goat's milk is lighter and forms less mucus.

Buttermilk can be taken with meals, as it stimulates digestion.

Fresh cheeses like ricotta and cottage cheese are easier to digest than hard, matured cheese or heavy creamy cheeses (such as brie) that create mucus. They're best enjoyed with black pepper to stimulate agni. Goat's cheese and feta are fine in moderation.

SPICES

Cumin, coriander, fennel, ginger, and saffron. These are the best for balancing the doṣa, increasing agni. They can be used liberally with turmeric, cinnamon, cardamom, mustard seeds, and fresh herbs (particularly fresh coriander). Black pepper, cloves, and garlic are heating and to be used more moderately.

Asafetida reduces vata and should be added when cooking pulses, cabbage, and beans to reduce their gas-producing properties. It is very heating so add only a pinch while cooking.

Celtic sea salt or rock salt can be added to dishes. Cinnamon and cloves can be used more frequently in winter cooking.

Spices are important in food preparation—they act medicinally. The correct blend brings health and a greater sensory enjoyment of your food.

OIL
Sunflower oil, coconut, or olive oil.

Foods to Enjoy Occasionally

VEGETABLES
Cauliflower, Brussels sprouts, cabbage, peppers, broad beans, and potatoes.

PULSES
Chickpeas, chana dal, black-eyed peas, soy and kidney beans must all be soaked overnight and be well cooked.

TOFU
Tofu can be eaten occasionally and served with black pepper.

Foods to Avoid

WHEAT, MEAT, REFINED SUGAR
These foods decrease the digestive fire (agni) and produce mucus and toxins (aam). Of the types of meat, red meat (beef) especially creates these effects.

DEEP-FRIED FOODS
These are heavy to digest and increase vata.

SOUR FOODS

Tomatoes; all sour fruits, including plums, pineapples, lemons, grapefruit, strawberries, sour green grapes (sweet oranges such as mandarins and sweet pineapple may be enjoyed), vinegar, and hot spices, such as chilis, increase pitta and heat in the body, reducing digestive power.

FERMENTED FOOD AND DRINK

Alcohol, yogurt, cheese (especially old cheese), pickles, tempeh, miso, and foods containing yeast, such as marmite, vegemite, and soy sauce. All fermented foods are sour in nature and therefore have pitta-increasing qualities. Whenever there is too much pitta and heat in the intestines, fermentation is increased, resulting in gas and decreased digestive (assimilation) capacity.

Yogurt is both sour and heating; this creates blocks in the subtle channels (nādis) of the body. When eaten, it's best taken mixed with water, adding cumin or ginger as an antidote to the congestive, mucus-forming properties.

ICE-COLD FOOD AND DRINKS

Ice cold drinks and food immediately dampen and lower the digestive fire.

PROCESSED FOOD

Processed food, canned food, microwavable food, stale and leftover food. These have little nutritional value and only serve to fill an empty space in the tummy. These foods deplete the digestive fire and take lots of energy to digest. Thus, these foods create an accumulation of sludge and excess gases and fluid in the body.

Energy-Rich Ayu Recipes

· · · · · · · · · · · ·

HERE ARE A few simple, nourishing dishes recommended to support your digestion. Enjoy.

Sāttvic Kichadi

1 cup basmati rice
½ cup yellow mung beans
3 to 5 cups water
1 Tbsp ghee
1 tsp each ground turmeric, cumin, coriander
1 pinch asafetida*
1 Tbsp fresh ginger, chopped, or 1 tsp ground ginger
2 cardamom pods, bruised
½ tsp Celtic sea salt or salt
½ tsp mustard seeds (optional)
Shredded coconut and chopped coriander, to taste

Wash the mung beans and rice together. Cook immediately in a pressure cooker, or soak for fifteen to thirty minutes. Discard the soaking liquid and re-rinse.

Heat the ghee in a large saucepan, add the spices and ginger. Sauté lightly, adding mung beans and rice, stirring to coat for greater absorption of the spices. Add three cups of water, or up to five for a soupier consistency. Add the cardamom pods, salt, and mustard seeds. Bring the ingredients to a boil and cook until the individual grains of rice are completely soft.

Serve with extra ghee. Garnish with shredded coconut and freshly chopped coriander.

*Available at health-food stores and Asian grocers.

(Serves 2 to 3)

Magic Mung Soup

1 cup whole green mung beans
1 Tbsp ghee
1 small onion, finely chopped (optional)
1 Tbsp fresh ginger, grated or finely chopped
1 tsp each ground turmeric, cumin, coriander, fennel, black pepper
1 pinch asafetida
1 bay leaf
6 to 8 cups water
Celtic sea salt or salt, to taste
Fresh coriander, to taste

Wash the mung beans. Soak for thirty minutes or overnight. Discard the soaking liquid and rinse the beans.

Heat the ghee in a large saucepan. Add the onion, ginger, and spices. Sauté lightly, then add mung beans and stir to coat for greater absorption of the spices. Add water and salt. Bring to a boil and cook until the mung beans are completely soft.

Add black pepper to taste and serve with extra ghee. Garnish with freshly chopped coriander.

When using this as a cleansing food, use more liquid for a soupy texture rather than that of a thick stew.

(Serves 4)

Daily Energy-Rich Drink

This drink, in itself, can be more than enough food and nourishing substance for many to begin the day. You can adjust the volume of water to get the consistency you best like or substitute the cardamom pods for ground cardamom or fennel. You may also add a dried fig for extra calcium or apricots that don't contain sulfur to build iron. This energy-rich drink is absolute gold for building sustenance to be a modern woman. It's a highly nutritious drink, high in iron, potassium (which fosters the uptake of calcium), protein, and B-group vitamins. It increases digestion and energy, and gives strength.

4 dates, or 1 fresh Medjool date
6 almonds
2 cardamom pods
½ tsp fennel seeds

Soak the ingredients in ⅔ cup water, overnight. In the morning, blend and drink before eating breakfast.

(Serves 1)

Ginger Tea

1 1-inch piece ginger, grated or finely sliced
3 cups water

In a saucepan, bring ingredients to a boil and gently simmer for ten minutes. Pour the tea into a thermos to keep it hot and sip throughout the day.

Alternatively, combine a few slices of fresh ginger and two cups of boiling water in a tea pot. Steep for five to ten minutes and drink.

Or add ½ tsp ginger powder to one cup of boiling water and drink.

Metabolic Spice Tea

1 tsp each ground cumin, coriander, and ginger
3 cups water

In a saucepan, combine ingredients, stir, and bring to a boil. Gently simmer for ten minutes before serving. Pour the tea into a thermos to keep it hot and sip throughout the day.

Self-Care Practices

· · · · · · · · · · · ·

THE FOLLOWING SELF-CARE practices are to establish nourishing rest-repair digestive health of the parasympathetic nervous system:

- Establish a regular meditation practice. A daily practice is ideal. When you establish yourself in the regular practice of meditation, it builds the muscle of being able to rest, repair, and replenish. Then it becomes a more familiar way of being and helps you navigate life responsively as opposed to being in the constantly reactive fight-flight-freeze mode. You are able to observe more clearly. Your faculty of perception becomes more refined as your awareness expands. For wellness, this keeps your inner garden maintained and conditions ripe to flourish in the elements. Be realistic about the time you can dedicate this. Keep it do-able. That means, if you can give it ten minutes a day to start, wonderful! Do it! Ways of meditating can include mantra japa, yoga nidra, restorative yoga, yin yoga, tai chi, sitting for guidance and journaling.

- Get good quality sleep.

- Stay well hydrated and regularly cleanse to clear accumulated toxins and inflammation, which are created by the stress hormones adrenaline and cortisol.

- Drink pure, clean water. Drinking fresh vegetable juices also is a great way to rest-repair digestive health. You can make veggie juice a combination of beetroot, carrot, apple, and celery. You may add small knob of fresh ginger, turmeric, and other seasonal veggies, including spinach and pomegranate.

- Drink one teaspoon of ghee mixed in hot water in the morning before tea/coffee/food to pacify internal stress and the nervous system.

- Do abhyanga, or self-oil massage. Before a bath or shower, massage your body with warm sesame oil (or almond oil). In particular, massage first the soles of the feet (which have thousands of nerve dendrites) and the lower abdomen. This keeps the body strengthened, pacified, and it is nourishment for nervous system.

- Take foot baths with lemon, lavender, or Epsom salts.

- Practice prāṇāyāma. This Sanskrit word means extension of the breath, prāṇā. When we deliberately, consciously work with our breath, we are able to influence the state of our mind and even our hormonal balance rapidly. A full, deep, relaxed breath is the main aim of breathing exercises, or prāṇāyāma. Breathing is something we can cultivate to do well constantly throughout each day. It is not only to be focused on while meditating, doing yoga, or exercising.

Homemade Pain Relievers

· · · · · · · · · · · · ·

THE FOLLOWING ARE homemade pain relievers recommended by Ayurveda.

General Premenstrual Discomfort

¼ cup ground ginger
2 Tbsp ground fenugreek
2 Tbsp ghee
⅓ cup jaggery or coconut sugar

Combine ingredients and mix well together. Roll into balls half an inch in diameter. Eat one each morning on an empty stomach. Seven days before menstruation is due, eat two a day.

Abdominal Pain

½ tsp ground dill seed
¼ tsp ground ginger
¼ tsp ground ajwain (wild celery seed)

1 pinch asafetida
1 tsp ground cumin
1 tsp jaggery
¾ cup water
1 tsp aloe vera juice

Combine ingredients in a saucepan and simmer for few minutes. Filter and drink twice a day, particularly ten days before the first day of menstruation and during menstruation.

Bloating and Premenstrual Symptoms

1 tsp ground cumin
½ tsp ground fennel
¼ tsp ground ajwain
1 pinch asafetida
1 tsp black salt (sanchal), if available
½ cup water

Mix ingredients together and simmer for a few minutes. Filter and drink daily.

Enrichment Activities

. . . .

Enrichment Activity #1:
Contemplate Digestion

Take three minutes to reflect on your digestion today. Yes, right now! How do you feel you are digesting your life, the food you eat, all your feelings and thoughts, all your challenges and stressors, your needs, all your joy and love, your dreams and hopes, your aspirations, this day? *Everything* that you are feeling this very day.

I invite you to get comfortable, cozy, close your eyes and reflect on this for three minutes. Then, when you have completed your reflection, you are invited to journal with pen and paper (preferably with hand and ink to the page instead of fingers on a keyboard, typing). Please write for another three minutes about whatever comes up, whatever comes to you.

Now, take another minute and imagine what your life would be like with robust, hearty digestion. How would this look? How would this feel for you?

Enrichment Activity #2:
Contemplate Digestion of Life

In your own words and with your own understanding write a few lines about what good digestion of life means to you.

Enrichment Activity #3:
Review General Ayurvedic Diet Guidelines

Read through the general Ayurvedic diet guidelines (appendix B). Write a list of things you are doing *now* that support your digestion.

Write a list of things that you can do that will support your digestion.

Write a brief list of things you can change that will support your digestion.

Enrichment Activity #4:
Establish Daily Rhythms

For the next seven days you are invited to practice the following daily routines:

- Get up at the same time each morning. Ideally between 5 a.m. and 7 a.m. (If you have been working late, are unwell, or are having broken sleep to care for others, you can have a reprieve and sleep until 8 a.m.!)

- Be outdoors in the elements each morning for ten to twenty minutes, either walking, sitting, meditating, doing yoga, or whatever activity calls you. The point of this pattern is to receive the essence and rhythm of the light from the rising sun at this time of day.

- Eat your meals at a similar time each day. Lunch between noon and 1 p.m. is ideal. If your usual lunch time to eat is 2 p.m. that is fine. However, keep it at that time consistently for this coming week. And, if you usually take your lunch at noon then ensure that this is consistent and you do not skip the meal or eat at 3 p.m.

- Go to bed at 10 p.m. and lights out 10:30 p.m. for the next week. If you go to bed earlier, that is even better! Please do not feel you have to stay up until 10 p.m. Remember, dear one, that your metabolic activity between 10 p.m. and 2 a.m. is cleansing your cells and it's cleaning time in your liver. This means more glowing vitality in your skin. This also supports you to be up earlier and take in the morning light before you commence the tasks of your busy day.

Enrichment Activity #5:
Follow the Checklist for Good Sleep

For the next week you are asked to focus on cultivating habits conducive for good sleep. You are invited to keep a journal and write down the steps you have taken to support your sleep, along with your observations of your sleep and energy experiences throughout the week. Follow the steps in Enrichment Activity #3, except focus habits that support sleep.

- Refrain from any kind of screen time activity for thirty minutes before sleep. This includes your phone. If your phone is used as an alarm, switch to airplane mode when you go to bed. If you do not need your phone as an alarm, then do not keep it in your bedroom overnight while you sleep.

- Ensure any electronic devices in the room are switched off at the wall. Better still, remove any screens from your bedroom.

- Draw your curtains and do what you can to ensure your room is as quiet and dark as possible. Use eye mask if your room is affected by light from street lamps and the like.

- If you can tolerate cow's milk, drink a small cup of hot milk (preferably organic, unhomogenized) spiced with turmeric, cinnamon, ginger, fennel and cardamom before bed. (This is not recommended if you have flu, cold, or fever.)

- Write a list of things you are grateful for in your day. A kind word, gesture, thought, your wellness, your golden mind, your warm cozy bed, your hot water bottle, your friends, your garden....

- When you go to bed lie on your left side for the first five to ten minutes, then move to your chosen position for sleep. This encourages vata to move in it's direct path, translating to better digestive processes, mental activity, and good sleep.

- Starting from your current moment, review your day backwards. You are simply observing without judgment or trying to find solutions. This is beginning the process of mentally digesting your day and encourages greater sleep easing the task of your body to digest all your experiences passively for you.

Enrichment Activity #6:
Practice Reflective Listening

This exercise is to prepare yourself inwardly to cleanse of any accumulation that prevents you from hearing the sound of your own unique self. You may ask following questions of yourself and reflect on what you hear.

These are questions and answers, posed by the great Sufi musician and mystic Hazrat Inayat Khan in *The Mysticism of Sound and Music*: How does one find the sound of one's key note once it is lost? It is never lost altogether, but only hidden from one's view. It is just the same when people say a person has lost his soul. The person is the soul. How, then, can one lose one's soul?

The key note is there. One must discover it. One must find it. You must begin from the first truth.

Has not every nerve its own sound? Yes, it has its own vibration. You may call it sound.

Beautiful woman, how do you recognize this sound? How do you hear this sound in the depths of your being?

To hear this sound, you cleanse. You clear the path.

Enrichment Activity #7:
Reflect on Nourishment

Take a quiet, reflective moment in your day. You are invited to create the gentle space to sit and reflect on all the nourishing substance you feed yourself daily:

- Contemplate, what is the essence of this?

- What does nourishment mean to you?

- What are you really feeding?

- What purpose is your nourishment serving in your life?

Write, unedited, about what comes up for you. Simply scribe *whatever* comes through you to the page.

Next ask yourself the following questions:

- What nourishment do I need this day?

- What does nourishment look like to me this day? You may ask for guidance from your higher self or a God of your understanding, whatever you relate to.

Write in your journal about what comes up for you. Be open to what comes to you and simply write and observe, without judgement or the need for perfection! You are already whole and complete.

Enrichment Activity #8:
Nourish with Gratitude

Make a list of all the things you are grateful for that have nourished you this day. It may be the fresh, seasonal food you have eaten or been served. The cup of tea, the scone with jam *and* cream! It may have been a quiet walk or a rigorous row in a boat. It may have been a quote of inspiration you read at the local gas station. It may have been a gesture of warmth and kindness from a complete stranger or perhaps a cuddle from your pet on your lap. It may have been sitting to rest and catch your breath or being so moved by the beauty of the setting sun. It may have been the glass of fresh water that quenched your thirst. The coziness of your socks. The fresh air you breathe.

Fill yourself with the nourishment of gratitude.

Enrichment Activity #9:
Examine the Guṇas at Play in You

This mental constitution chart is designed to examine yourself and understand a little more about the quality of your mind and the guṇas.

This chart is for yourself. It is not about having the most sāttvic qualities for your answers but really to gain an understanding of the type of quality of mind you are experiencing in your life and the impact of this on your vitality and life energy. There are no right or wrong answers in this exercise. You are encouraged to complete this chart reflectively, honestly, and objectively. This is the whole point of the activity, to cultivate your awareness of your great self! You may ask a friend or partner to do this with you. They will be more objective about you than you may be about yourself.

MENTAL CONSTITUTION CHART

Diet	vegetarian	some meat	heavy meat diet
Alcohol, drugs and stimulants	never	occasionally	frequently
Sensory impressions	calm, gentle	mixed	disturbed
Sleep requirements	little	moderate	high
Sensory impressions	calm, gentle	mixed	disturbed
Control of senses	good	moderate	weak
Speech	calm, soothing, peaceful	agitated	dull
Cleanliness	high	moderate	low
Life's work	selfless	for personal goals	lazy
Anger	rarely	sometimes	frequently
Fear	rarely	sometimes	frequently
Greed	little	some	a lot
Envy	little	some	a lot
Desire	little	some	a lot
Pride	modest	some ego	quite vain
Depression	never	sometimes	frequently
Love	universal	personal	lacking
Violent behavior	never	sometimes	frequently
Attachment to money	little	some	a lot
Attachment to material things	little	some	a lot
Contentment	mostly	sometimes	rarely
Forgiveness	easily forgiving	forgiving with effort	holds grudges long term

Concentration and focus	good	moderate	poor
Memory	good	moderate	poor
Willpower	strong	variable	weak
Truthfulness	always	much of the time	not often
Ease	generally	sometimes	not often
Peace of Mind	generally	sometimes	not often
Creativity	high	moderate	low
Spiritually orientated study	daily	occasionally	never
Prayer, mantra	daily	occasionally	never
Meditation	daily	occasionally	never
Community service/ charity	much	some	none
Acts of self-care	daily	occasionally	never
TOTAL	**SĀTTVA**	**RĀJAS**	**TĀMAS**

Enrichment Activity #10:
Do the Miraculous Mung Soup Cleanse

You are invited to do a one-day mung soup cleanse. Plan and prepare yourself. Is the cleanse timely? Do you have the ingredients on hand to prepare your soup and have it ready to eat before breakfast on the day of your cleanse?

I encourage you to prepare the soup the evening before so that you can eat it for breakfast and take a thermos of soup for lunch that day. No vegetables, fruit, nuts, cheese, crackers, alcohol, or juices. Only soup. As much as you want, but only soup.

Keep a journal during your cleanse. What did the cleanse look and feel like for you? Did any resistance come up, and what was it?

How was your energy throughout the day? Were you feeling steady, vital, sluggish, tired, excited, connected, angry; did you have a headache? How did your gut feel? How did you sleep on the day of your cleanse?

It is best to avoid caffeinated drinks on cleansing day. However, if you are a regular coffee drinker consider this when planning your cleansing day because you may feel headache, dullness, nausea, or even vomiting.

If it feels too difficult to cleanse without your coffee or tea, then with compassion I would say a cleanse with one coffee or tea is better than no cleanse at all! You can use your own discernment here.

Drink ginger tea throughout your day or metabolic spice tea, which converts aam into energy. (See appendix C.) You may also drink tulsi (holy basil) tea.

On your cleansing day, I recommend you go to bed early. If you are hungry, looking for food or chocolate, then pat yourself on the back, acknowledge what a great effort you have made, and swiftly go to bed! Call it a day well lived.

I find that when I'm cleansing, my energy levels are steadier throughout the day, but I'm ready for bed earlier. This is something I really honor and I go to bed at 9 p.m. or by 10 p.m. I tuck myself in bed and read or journal.

Notes on the Transliteration and Pronunciation of Sanskrit

· · · · · · · · · · · ·

THE TRANSLITERATION OF Sankrit, Hindi, or Marathi in the Sanskrit terms and mantras in this book may not be exact in phonetic transcription, but can be used this way as the Devanāgarī script correlates to the sounds. This appendix is offered as an explanation of the diacritical marks and general guide to Sanskrit pronunciation.

Vowels
· · · · · · · · · ·

Vowels can be short or long. The long vowels are indicated by a line above. A long vowel is held for twice as long as a short one. That means *ā* is held for the length of time it would take to pronounce two *a*'s.

a as in cup, gut	*ā* as in father, balm
i as in sit, grit	*ī* as in clean, seen
u as in foot, put	*ū* as in food, broom
e as in play, or French les	*o* as in French beau

ai as in hay   au as in now, bough
ṛ as in Kṛsna

Consonants

k as in kaftan, kitten   c as in much, chop
t, d, n are pronounced with tip of tongue lightly touching spot at top
back of front teeth, as in teeth, dinner, nice.
ṭ, ḍ, ṇ are pronounced with tip of tongue curling back slightly to
touch tiny cave in roof of mouth.
ñ as in onion, señor
ś as in shiny, shave, shimmer
ṣ as in ssssssssshhhhhhh with tip of tongue touching roof of mouth,
slightly curled back like above ṭ, as in Kṛsna, Aṣtanga.

When consonants are followed by an h, they are aspirated: Kh as
in cough.
ḥ at the end of a word means there's a slight aspiration that echoes
the previous vowel.

Pronouncing the Mantras

There are three main elements to practice when pronouncing Sanskrit mantras:
1. the time taken to pronounce the letter
2. the placement of the tongue
3. the aspiration (or unaspiration) with the letter
The mātrā is the measurement of time for the duration of the
vowel. One count is about the time it takes to snap your fingers.
Short vowels are one count, and long vowels are two counts.

As consonants do not appear without a vowel, this measurement
is applied generally to the vowels.

Importance is given to the emphasis on vowel duration because
the alternation of the length of one letter can completely change the
meaning of the Sanskrit word.

The placement and position of the tongue is important because this changes the pronunciation of the letter. This, too, can change the meaning of the word.

There are five positions of the tongue which move the sound from guttural in the throat to the lips.

These five tongue positions are called *guttural, palatal, cerebral, dental,* and *labial.*

In Sanskrit words, the distinction between aspirated and unaspirated consonants also can change the meaning of the word.

Examples of aspirated consonants are:

About. The *b* is unaspirated. The *t* is aspirated.

Make. The *m* is unaspirated. The *k* is aspirated.

Apple. The *p* is unaspirated.

Push. The *p* is aspirated.

In Sanskrit, a unaspirated consonant has no breath with it. An aspirated consonant is with breath.

Guide to Diacritical Marks

ā a line over the vowel means it's long and is held for two counts.

ḍ a dot under a letter (except *ḥ*) means it's pronounced from the cerebral position, with the tongue curled slightly up and touching the little "cave" in the roof of the mouth.

ñ a tilde over the letter indicates a nasal sound with tension back of the palate. Pronounced like "*nya.*"

aḥ *ḥ* is pronounced with slight aspiration. When at end of sentence there is an echo of the preceding vowel. Thus, when placed at end of sentence *namaḥ* is pronounced "*namaha.*"

ṅ a dot above an *n* means it is pronounced "*ng.*"

ṁ a dot above an *m* means it's an *anusvara*. The tongue lightly touches the roof of the mouth and it's an inward dissolving sound.

ś an *s* with acute accent is pronounced as "*sh.*"

Glossary

. . . .

Aam (Ama): Metabolic sludge (toxins) created by incomplete digestion.

Abhyanga: Self-massage with oil.

Agni: Digestive fire; the fire of metabolism.

Ākāśa: Ether.

Anusvāra: The after sound of resonance following a vowel (ṁ or sometimes written as ṃ).

Apāna vāyu: The downward moving aspect of prāṇa vāyu (air). Moves from navel to perineum and is responsible for elimination and reproductive function.

Asafetida: A resin used therapeutically in cooking.

Āsana: A physical posture.

Asthi: Tissue of bone.

Auṁ: A sacred mantra. The primordial sound of the cosmos. Consciousness embodied in the form of pulsating sound.

Bīja: Seed.

Buddhi: Discriminating aspect of the mind. Intelligence.

Cakra: Energy center.

Caraka Saṃhitā: A classic Sanskrit text on Ayurveda.

Cit (citta): Mental field of consciousness.

Dhara: Stream or current of liquid.

Dhātu: Tissue.

Dośa: Governing force or biological humor of Ayurveda.

Ekāgracitta: One-pointed focus.

Gaṅgā: The most sacred river in India, revered as a goddess.

Guṇa: Quality of nature. In Ayurveda: sāttva, rājas, and tamas.

Hṛidaya: Heart.

Jala: Water.

Kapha: Governing force of cohesion. Biological earth/water humor.

Karma: Any action, physical or mental. The fruition of an action arising from desire.

Kuṇḍalinī: The divine power or primordial energy. The extremely subtle force that lays coiled at the base of the spine (in the base cakra) in each human.

Lakṣmi: The goddess who embodies abundance, prosperity, beauty, grace, vitality. Also called Śrī.

Majja: Tissue of bone marrow, nerve.

Māmsa: Tissue of muscle.

Manas: The mind. That which receives information from the sense organs.

Mantra: Sacred sounds invested with the power to purify and transform the awareness of the one who repeats them.

Mantra puruṣa: The subtle sound body.

Marma: Energy point in the body.

Marma chikitsa: Energy-point treatment.

Medha: Fat (adipose) tissue.

Nāda: Inner sound.

Nāda yoga: The yoga of sound.

Nāḍi: Pulse, channel.

Ojas: Pure vital essence.

Panchakarma: Ayurvedic deep therapeutic cleansing and detoxification program of mind, body, and emotions.

Pitta: Governing force of energy. Biological fire humor.

Prakṛti: Inherent physiological constitution.

Prāṇa: Life force; vital breath.

Prāṇāyāma: Controlled breathing exercises and practices.

Pṛthvī: Earth.

Pūrṇam: Full, whole, complete.

Puruṣa: The innermost self, the higher self.

Rājas: One of the three guṇas: the quality of energy, agitation.

Rakta: Tissue of blood.

Rasa: Tissue of plasma, lymph. Also flavor, essence.

Rumi, Jalal Al-Din Muhammad (1207–1273): Ecstatic poet of the Sūfi tradition.

Śakti: Power, energy. Power of the divine goddess.

Sanskrit: Ancient language of India. Considered to be the language of the gods.

Sarasvāti: Goddess of learning, wisdom, arts.

Sāttva: One of the three guṇas: the quality of light, harmony, purity.

Śiva Saṃhitā: A sacred Sanskrit text on yoga.

śukra: Reproductive tissue.

Suśruta Saṃhitā: A classic Sanskrit text on Ayurvedic medicine and surgery.

Tāmas: One of the guṇas: the quality of inertia, dullness, darkness.

Tantra: An ancient universal science and culture dealing with the transition of human nature at its present stage of evolution to a transcendental level of awareness and knowledge. Teachings and techniques of energetic yoga practices.

Ujjayi: A controlled breathing technique.

Vaca oil: Medicated castor oil with bitter herbs.

Vastu: Vedic science of architecture and direction.

Vata: Governing force of motion. Biological air humor.

Veda: Sacred knowledge.

Vikṛti: Imbalanced state. Deviation from nature.

Yaṁ: Bīja mantra for the heart cakra and rasa dhātu, lymph, and plasma.

Yoga: Specific practices of body, subtle body, and mind aimed at self-knowledge. The goal is union with Self.

Yoga āsana: A physical yoga posture.

References

Desikachar, T.K.V. *The Heart of Yoga: Developing a Personal Practice.* Rochester, Vermont: Inner Traditions, 1995.

Frawley, David. *Ayurveda and the Mind: The Healing of Consciousness.* Twin Lakes, Wisconsin: Lotus Press, 1996.

———. *Mantra Yoga and Primal Sound: Secret of Seed (Bija) Mantras.* Twin Lakes, Wisconsin: Lotus Press, 2010.

Helmut-Hemmerich, Fritz. *Handbook of Anthroposophic Gynecology.* Spring Valley, New York: Mercury Press, 2007.

Hersey, Baird, and Sri Krishna Das. *The Practice of Nada Yoga: Meditation on the Inner Sacred Sound.* Rochester, Vermont: Inner Traditions, 2014.

Khan, Hazrat Inayat. *The Mysticism of Sound and Music: The Sufi Teaching of Hazrat Inayat Khan.* Boston: Shambhala Dragon Editions, 1991.

König, Karl. *A Living Physiology: Lectures and Essays.* Camphill: Camphill Books, 2006.

Robertson, Caroline. *Vastu Shastra: The Indian Counterpart to Feng Shui.* Sydney: Lansdowne, 2000.

Roche, Lorin. *The Radiance Sutras: 112 Gateways to the Yoga of Wonder and Delight.* Boulder: Sounds True, 2014.

Steiner, Rudolf. *Course for Young Doctors.* Chestnut Ridge, New York: Mercury Press, 1994.

———. The Healing Processes: Spirit, Nature, and Our Bodies. Great Barrington, Massachusetts: Steiner Press, 1999.

———. The Inner Nature of Music and the Experience of Tone. Milton: Mercury Press, 1983.

Svoboda, Robert. Ayurveda for Women: A Guide to Vitality and Health. Devon: David & Charles, 1999.

Welch, Claudia. Balance Your Hormones, Balance Your Life: Achieving Optimal Health and Wellness through Ayurveda, Chinese Medicine, and Western Science. Cambridge: Da Capo Lifelong Books, 2011.

Endnotes

. . . .

1. Dr. David Frawley, in chapter 3 of his book *Ayurveda and the Mind*, eloquently describes the guṇas.

2. For a most comprehensive resource on mantra, mantra yoga, and the use of mantra in modern life, I recommend you read Anandra George of True Freedom Coaching's free ebook, *Mantra Yoga*. It is a thorough, succinct, practical, and inspiring resource. Dr. David Frawley's book *Mantra and Primal Sound* is another deep reference on mantra and sacred Sanskrit syllables that I wholly recommend. Dr. Frawley says, "Mantra is the essence of the great yogic teaching as well as its primary practice."

About the Author

. . . .

DIPIKA DELMENICO is an Ayurvedic Medicine Practitioner, Anthroposophic Naturopath, Yoga of Sound teacher, international speaker, and author. She's practiced clinically for more than twenty years, treating thousands of patients globally with Ayurveda healing wisdom and mantra. Dipika's previous book is the bestseller *Shine Your Light*. She's the founder of The Radiant Woman wellness courses, Alchemy of Sound Programs, and Conscious Woman Rising.

Dipika works therapeutically with mantra and sacred sound as the original medicine, and medicine of our future. She is in service to the renewal of ancient healing mysteries and healing the divine feminine in each of us.

dipikadelmenico.com